EVERYDAY STRUGGLES

A Straightforward Comprehension of Self Improvement and
Cherishing Yourself and Tolerating Change

RAUL RUELAS

Contents

Introduction

Every day we struggle. We struggle with our relationships, our finances, our careers, and even our own selves. Sometimes it seems like all we ever do is struggle. It's as if we are pushing a huge boulder up a hill, and we are always just a step away from being squished. This boulder represents life and its many challenges such as stress, not loving yourself, or even change. And most of the time, we are never ready for these challenges.

Take change, for instance; every day, you are faced with it. Sometimes it's little things such as changing your usual seat on the bus. Other times it's something big, like dealing with job loss or the death of a loved one. In both instances, you have to deal with uncertainty but it's harder to bounce back in the case of losing your job or a loved one.

So what can you do? How can you prepare for life's challenges?

It's simple, take it a day at a time or, in this case, one challenge at a time. To help you do that, we will look at some crucial areas that you can work on to help you better face these challenges. The first chapter will look at self-love, what it is, what it looks like, its importance, the distinction between self-love and narcissism, and how to practice self-love. This chapter is crucial because a lot of us have a hard time loving and accepting ourselves for who we are. We live wearing masks that, if taken off, would reveal a lot of hurt, confusion, and lack of love.

After learning about self-love, we will delve into habits. After all, not loving yourself is a habit you might have, and we need to change it. However, changing habits takes a lot more than just deciding to change. It requires a lot of conscious effort and determination. You will only build better habits if you understand how they work and hack the system. That's what the chapters on habits will focus on—getting you well informed about your habits and how to build better ones.

Subsequent chapters will look into relationships and why they matter. Having healthy relationships is a crucial part of the new life you are trying to build, so make sure you pay close attention to that. We will also look at stress, overcoming failure, procrastination, and more, so read on.

Most people think the struggles they face in life are due to external factors and have nothing to do with them. However, this isn't entirely true. While there are things that are out of your control, there are those that you have power over. These include learning how to love and accept yourself, changing your habits, dealing with challenges, change, and failure, as well as learning to be content and happy. They make up over 90 percent of your life, meaning you have the power to change the outcomes.

Surviving these everyday struggles is not a race but a marathon. You have to learn how to pace yourself through the many steps you need to take to become a better you. Be honest about where you are in life and where you want to go and then take the steps towards changing your life. As you read on, remain open-minded, and you might learn a thing or two.

Happy reading!

ONE

The Power of Self-Love

"I'M NOT GOOD ENOUGH."

"I'll never make it."

We have all had these and other self-defeating thoughts at one point in our lives. We are our own worst judge, and we are pretty good at pointing out the negatives in our lives. But why do we do that? Why do we easily believe the most detrimental things about ourselves? Well, it all boils down to our minds. The human mind is a central issue; our thoughts are responsible for how our lives are. It's not about what you know but how you think that matters. This means that, despite knowing that you are capable of doing something or that you are worth it, you still convince yourself that you are lacking and don't deserve anything good in your life.

Pretty dark, huh? Well, your thoughts are that potent; they can influence your emotions, beliefs, habits, actions, and even your character. Did you know that you have anywhere between 12,000 to 60,000 thoughts in a day? That's about 2,500 to 3,300 thoughts an hour. Of these, 80 percent are negative, and 95 percent of the 80 percent are repetitive. This means that only about 20 percent of all the thoughts you have in a day are positive.

This basically means that we end up repeating the same negative thoughts more than the positive ones over and over during the day. Picture it this way, if you did something over 2,000 times an hour all day, every day, what effect would it have on you?

Think about that for a minute.

Here are some more interesting facts. Remember those negative thoughts you keep having all day about how you are not good enough or how you don't deserve good things? Well, 85 percent of the things you worry about never happen. For instance, if you are worried about not being good enough to get a job, there's an 85 percent chance that it doesn't matter. What about the 15 percent that's left? Well, that does happen, but it's not as bad as you think. You end up finding out you could easily handle it or you learn a valuable lesson.

So what does all this math say? About 97 percent of the worries you have are baseless because they are a result of unfounded pessimistic perception or a negative mindset. This negative mindset can affect your self-esteem, confidence, and what you think of yourself. So how can you change from this self-sabotaging state of mind to a more positive one? It's through self-love.

What is Self-Love?

Self-love is a state of appreciation of yourself or regarding yourself as worthy and prioritizing your own wellbeing and happiness. How you see yourself is how you see the world; if you aren't good enough, then neither will anyone or anything else be, and vice versa. Self-love is about having compassion and unconditionally accepting yourself. It means taking care of your needs before prioritizing those of others. Simply put, self-love is about viewing yourself as worthy, valuable, good, and deserving of love and happiness.

Sounds easy enough, right?

Yet, we all desperately fail at it. Self-love goes beyond eating a healthy diet or saying a hundred affirmations every day. It is about finding that missing piece of you, the part that makes everything fit into place. We are all miserably aware that something is missing within us. Think of things that would give you the power to continue your diet, get up and work out, or leave an abusive relationship. That missing piece is self-love.

If you don't love yourself, then you will always be looking for someone to love you. Sometimes you find someone to do it, but it's only a temporary fix because how can you expect someone else to love the parts of you that you don't even love yourself? Unable to love these parts of yourself, you seek validation and approval from others, often going to ridiculous lengths to get it. However, this only sets you up for more hurt because it encourages abandonment and rejection. If you cannot accept yourself as you are, you can't expect others to accept you. This lack of self-acceptance has you living in a constant state of fear—the fear of rejection.

Narcissism vs. Self-Love

Healthy self-love is a precarious balance between low self-esteem or a lack of self-love and grandiosity, which is an inflated, false self-love that's overcompensating for lacking true self-love. The latter can easily turn into narcissism if taken to the extreme. So what is the difference between true self-love and narcissism? While both involve loving oneself, the biggest difference between the two is how you treat others.

Self-love is about truly connecting with yourself and loving every part of you without making comparisons. It's about taking pride in your achievements and performance, while recognizing it's okay to feel uncertain at times. Narcissism, on the other hand, is the complete opposite. Narcissists often compare themselves to others to feel better. They are obsessed with looking the part instead of playing it, often seeking validation from others. Their world view is often black and white; you are either in or out.

Narcissism is about proving you are better than others and making sure that everybody sees it, while self-love is an authentic, honest appreciation for yourself. It is self-focused, meaning the only opinion that matters is yours, whereas narcissism is other-focused, meaning other people's opinion matters.

Self-Love Deficit Disorder (SLDD)

This disorder can be defined as an absence of self-love, which leads you to develop insecurities, which in turn, keep you from forming healthy relationships. Simply put, it's another way of defining codependency. People suffering from SLDD often have difficult and dysfunctional relationships because what they are looking for cannot be found in others. They form unhealthy attachments to those they love, often looking to them for validation and approval.

Individuals with SLDD develop the problems they have in stages. Stage one is the root cause of the problem—the attachment trauma. This can be growing up with a narcissistic parent who gave you conditional and judgmental love. This childhood trauma is often repressed, and as you grow up, you develop feelings of worthlessness and think you are unlovable. You think if your parents couldn't love you unconditionally, who will?

The second stage is where you develop a core sense of shame because of the distorted views you have about yourself. For instance, you might start thinking that you are only as good as the things you can do for others, or that you are only lovable to a certain point. These negative thoughts fan the flames of the distorted self-view you have and worsen your inner shame. This leads you to push others away and isolate yourself, feeding a pathological need for loneliness.

This is ironic because, despite pushing people away, you are incredibly lonely and desperately longing for love and affection. In this vulnerable emotional state, SLDD individuals are often drawn to narcissists who happily take advantage of them. Having found love, acceptance, and affection in the narcissist, you get temporary relief from the loneliness you feel. However, soon you find out that the narcissist you thought was going to save you is a difficult, often impossible person to be in a relationship with.

They lie, use, and manipulate you, giving you just enough love and affection that you feel compelled to stay. This results in an unhealthy addiction to the emotional abuse caused by the relationship. The final stage is SLDD. You become a selfless, compulsive caretaker who tries to control others into loving you.

What Does Self-Love Look Like?

You have probably heard it a lot of times before; you can't truly love someone until you love yourself, or you can't take care of someone else until you take care of yourself. That's the essence of self-love—you. It all starts with you. If you are not in a good place, with no balance, inner peace, or compassion, you are in no position to do your best loving or caring for someone.

Self-love is different for everybody because we all have different ways of taking care of ourselves. For instance, a high-performing student who failed a test might tell himself that it's okay, everybody fails sometimes, but it doesn't mean he is a failure. A mother who loses her temper and yells at her kid might tell herself that it's okay because it was just yelling and she can always apologize later.

For some, self-love is being kinder to themselves, prioritizing their needs, giving themselves a break from self-judgment, trusting themselves, setting healthy boundaries, being true to themselves, and forgiving themselves when they haven't lived up to their own standards. For others, self-love is a way of referring to self-care. With that in mind, self-love would be listening to our bodies, taking a break every once in a while, putting the phone down and having actual conversations with people, being nicer to yourself, and eating healthier but not judging yourself too harshly if you indulge every once in a while.

Why Self-Love Is Important

As stated before, self-love is a state of appreciation that grows from actions that support your physical, psychological, and spiritual growth.

By learning to value yourself as a human being deserving of love, joy, happiness, and peace, you can live a fulfilling life. Self-love is about accepting yourself for who you are at this very moment. It means accepting your emotions, both good and bad, for what they are and putting your physiological, emotional, and mental wellbeing first. There are a lot of benefits to it that include:

- **Helping prevent depression**

Low self-love comes with low self-compassion. Self-compassion is vital when it comes to protecting you from depression and its negative effects. Depression is an emotional state marked by feelings of low self-worth, low self-esteem, and feelings of guilt coupled with an inability to enjoy life. It can be caused by a variety of factors, such as worrying and stressing over things to a point where you see no hope. Research has shown that if you have low self-compassion, you are at a greater risk of avoiding your problems and ruminating over negative thoughts and feelings, which make it difficult to function normally.

Constantly going over negative thoughts such as how you aren't good enough or deserving of good things can trigger depression. However, self-compassion can act as a buffer between your fragile psyche and negative feelings such as self-judgment, self-isolation, and over-identification, all common in those suffering from depression. If you have higher self-compassion, you are generally less troubled by these symptoms. You are also less likely to judge yourself too harshly over your mistakes or isolate yourself from others. You can cope better with these issues than those with little to no self-compassion

- **Reducing stress**

With a healthy dose of self-love, you are less likely to stress over things that would normally be stressful. For instance, if you make a mistake, you understand that it's just a mistake; even though it might be bad, it's not the end of the world and you will recover from it. However, without self-love or self-compassion, this would seem like the end. Even a small mistake that's easily overlooked would feel like a mountain to you because you would overthink everything, mostly focusing on the negative.

- **Increasing Happiness**

If you love yourself, you are able to fully experience the joy and abundance that comes with life. Self-love frees you from the shackles of guilt, regret, and anger. This allows you to truly forgive and love yourself. You can form deeper relationships with others because you are living your truth. You don't depend on others to love or validate you, which means your happiness is self-made, not dependent on others.

Other benefits include a higher sense of optimism, which is amplified by your good mood and the positive effects self-love has. With this positive outlook, you are more optimistic about life and love. You become more outgoing, talkative, and full of energy. You are more motivated and willing to take the initiative, which shows you aren't afraid of failure. This opens you up to more learning experiences allowing you to gain a greater sense of wisdom.

This self-motivation and willingness to try new things is driven by an increased state of curiosity, a yearning to learn and explore. This is because you are no longer afraid of what might happen. You are confident in your abilities and ready to face any challenges. You also become more agreeable and conscientious.

The Key to Practicing Self-Love

When working on your acceptance and self-love, the first and most important step is determining who you are on those fronts. To assess your level of compassion, you can use this scale. It will help you think about how you tend to feel, think, and talk about yourself. This simple self-compassion scale was developed by Kristin Neff and is made up of 26 items categorized into 6 subcategories. You should respond based on how you typically act towards yourself during hard times.

· · ·

The 6 subcategories include:

1. Self-kindness. When you are going through a hard time, do you give yourself enough care and tenderness?
2. Self-judgment. Are intolerant or impatient about aspects of your personality that you don't like?
3. Common humanity. Whenever you feel inadequate, do you remind yourself that it's something a lot of people feel?
4. Isolation. Whenever you think of your inadequacies, do you feel detached from the rest of the world?
5. Mindfulness. Whenever you are feeling down, do you approach your feelings with openness and curiosity?
6. Over-identification. If you fail, do you become consumed by your feelings of inadequacy?

Each item is rated on a scale of 1 (almost never) to 5 (almost always) based on how you would typically react. Your cumulative score will give you an indication of where you are on the self-compassion scale. Once you know where you are, you can determine where you want to go and the best way to get there.

On your journey of self-love, the most crucial thing is overcoming your inner self-critic. Self-criticism is something a lot of people suffer from; however, we tend to overlook it. The way you talk to yourself plays a crucial role in your wellbeing; however, this can be fixed. As we continue, you have to remember that how you perceive yourself is never in an objective manner. We all have our own filters and perceptions that color our view of the world.

As you grow, you are conditioned by the people around you, often modeling your behavior and thought patterns after your caretakers. You are likely to adopt the same values that your caretakers live by. That's why if you had a narcissistic parent who rarely showed you love, you would have a hard time loving yourself. Values are a collection of guiding principles that help you decide what's right and wrong. They are a subconscious scoring system through which we assess others and ourselves in terms of worth and ideals. For example, responsibility and openness can strengthen relationships and improve wellbeing, as well as creativity.

Your subjective and self-critical views of whether you live up to these values can significantly impact your self-worth in the long run. This, in turn, determines the voices in your head that can either be supportive or destructive. What you must understand is that these perceptions affect and influence your behavior. Negative self-perception adversely affects your self-treatment, forcing you to prevent rather than promote your happiness and wellbeing.

How to Practice Self-Love and Make Peace with Your Inner Critic

It's natural to generally hide your shortcomings, whether real or not, in order to maintain your positive self-image. With a bit of self-love and compassion, you can increase your knowledge and clarity about your limitations. So how do you make peace with your inner critic? Here are a few ways you can do this while practicing self-love.

1. Forgive yourself

The first step is forgiving yourself for your mistakes. You are not perfect, so why hold yourself to unrealistic expectations? Failure is inevitable and part of the growth process. You are valued by others for who you are, not for your lack of flaws. So, understand that you don't need to be a certain way to be worthy of love. You need to become aware of the times you get a sense of self-worth from performance or perceived perfection.

A simple way to remind yourself you are worthy even when it doesn't feel like it is leaving little sticky notes on your fridge, your desk, or your wallet with a loving message reminding you to be kind to yourself. There's no value in punishing yourself for your mistakes. Forgive yourself, let it go, and learn from it.

2. Adopt a growth mindset

Our mindsets can greatly affect our wellbeing. If you have a fixed mindset, you have a hard time accepting failure, loving yourself, or facing challenges. However, with a growth mindset, you embrace change and view failure as a learning opportunity because you understand your failures don't define you. Whenever you find yourself negatively criticizing yourself or comparing yourself to others rather than seeing your own merits, try and draw inspiration from them. Don't let the success of others intimidate or threaten you; instead, let it be a learning opportunity and a chance to better yourself.

3. Be grateful

Gratitude is a strong emotion that can do wonders for your happiness levels and wellbeing. Instead of getting hung up wishing for what we don't have, there's strength in appreciating what you have at the moment. By focusing on your blessings, you actually learn that you have a lot going for yourself and can use a gentler, more loving inner voice. You can try keeping a gratitude journal, volunteering, practicing mindfulness, and taking gratitude walks. If you are having a hard time finding something to be grateful for, spend time with your loved ones or make a compliment.

4. Use releasing statements

You might not be a fan of using positive affirmations because they don't feel natural or don't quite touch your inner subconscious critic. In such cases, you can use releasing statements. They are mini-exercises in self-forgiveness that tap into the concept of detached non-judgment often employed when practicing mindfulness. Whenever you find yourself having negative thoughts, such as you are an idiot for not getting something right, turn it around and release yourself from feeling bad by saying it's okay to get upset.

5. Find the right generosity level for you

There are three reciprocity styles—being a giver, taker, and matcher. Givers are overly generous, which is a great way to employ compassion. However, their selfless giving can lead them to ignore their own needs. As a giver, for generosity to work and favor your wellbeing, it shouldn't be completely selfless. Before attending to the needs of others, you have to be aware of your own needs. Basically, this means taking care of yourself as you would take care of others.

By consciously tapping into caregiving and directing it towards yourself, you release oxytocin, a feel-good hormone that has several benefits. Afterwards, consciously choose who you want to give your generosity. Picking the right person to offer your generosity ensures you don't get sucked into a narcissistic web of deceit. Secondly, assess the resources you have available and the energy you have to do all this.

Remember to always have fun while being generous, see the difference between being selfless and being used, and don't forget to give back to yourself. While doing good to others makes us feel good, it doesn't mean we can't be good to ourselves.

6. Practice mindfulness

Mindfulness is a great way to center yourself in the moment. It is a core tenet of self-love and a great way to lessen self-judgment. Mindfulness is being aware of what's happening in the moment without judging or labeling it. It's about allowing what you are thinking or feeling to have its moment rather than shutting it down or hiding it. Allow it to come, acknowledge it, and then, without any judgment or attachment, let it go. Mindfulness goes hand in hand with other relaxation techniques such as meditation, yoga, and even exercising.

7. Regain your perspective

Whenever you find yourself being too harsh or judgmental of yourself, zoom out and remind yourself of everything you have going for you. Rather than focusing on this one bad moment, zoom out and see the bigger picture. There are several ways you can zoom out:

- Let go of outside validation—a lot of negative thinking stems from how we think of ourselves. If you beat yourself up over your weight, a lot of the pressure comes from societal influences that state you should look a certain way. However,

if you choose to let go of this societal pressure and accept
your body the way it is, you will be happier.
- Reach out to others—this might seem counterintuitive to the
  first point but hear me out. This isn't about looking for
  validation, but rather putting your feelings in context. By
  talking to others, you are able to realize that you are not the
  only one in pain. Connecting with others is an important part
  of reaffirming your sense of connectedness, seeing the bigger
  picture, and resolving your perceived problems, while
  building social networks that promote your wellbeing.

Remember, you are always worthy of love, especially from yourself. Be
mindful of the difficult emotions you experience, forgive yourself for
being human, and see the bigger picture and identify how you can do
better next time. The main takeaway is to accept yourself. You are
perfectly imperfect, and that's perfectly fine.

It is important to note that:

- Most of your thoughts will be negative; thus, changing even a
  small number of these thoughts can have a serious positive
  effect on your life.
- You cannot stop all the negative thoughts you have. The
  point of altering your thought patterns isn't to eliminate all
  negative thoughts but rather to raise your awareness of the
  presence of negative thought patterns. From there, you can
  work on reducing the ways and times you disempower
  yourself.
- Most problems stem from negative thinking. We have already
  established the power that your thoughts have. Problems or
  errors in thinking arise because we make our own
  interpretations of events and emotions we feel in our lives.
  This misinterpretation can lead to self-inflicted pain when
  you accept these negative thoughts.
- You do not have to accept your negative thought patterns
  because research has shown that with a positive, healthy
  thought process, you can challenge and dispel these thoughts

and beliefs. You can find alternative explanations of the beliefs you have adopted. It is not about tricking yourself into believing that everything is great, but rather developing a more realistic view you can learn from.

- It is your reactions or how you handle your thoughts that matters. You must accept that a lot of the things that happen will be out of your control, but you can manage your reactions to these events. For instance, do you view failure as a roadblock or a learning opportunity? It is not objective events that determine your success but rather how you handle them.

TWO

How Your Habits Shape Your Identity

A HABIT IS a set of intuitive, unconscious thoughts, behaviors, and emotions that you have acquired through repetition. This is when you do something so many times your body goes into autopilot mode. For instance, every morning when you wake up, you probably have a cup of coffee. You have done this for the longest time that it's automatic now: wake up, coffee. This is a habit.

If you are to undergo any genuine attempt to change yourself, you need to take a good, long look at your habits. We develop habits to help us navigate the world and we can be aware of them or not. Thanks to the basal ganglia, these behaviors are automatic, much like blinking, and they help us meet our daily needs more efficiently. However, because these habits are so deeply ingrained in us, even if a habit is bad, it can be difficult to break. Knowing how habits are formed is the first step, if any real effort is to be made to dismantle and replace them.

Habits can be good or bad. Having coffee first thing in the morning, taking a run, going to the gym, hard work, reading, writing, meditation, dishonesty, escapism, or buckling your seatbelt are all examples of habits. Most of us have habits we don't even pay any attention to. For example, we brush our teeth at night while on autopilot. This is a beneficial habit, so we don't need to worry about it, but what about all those negative habits that are also automatic or on autopilot?

Your life is a summation of your habits. How content or miserable you are, whether you are in shape or not, and how successful or unsuccessful you are depends on your habits. What you repeatedly do, or spend time thinking about every day, ultimately forms your personality, beliefs, and personhood. Think about that for a minute. It's not your spouse's fault that you're not happy at home or your boss' fault that you hate your job; it's all your fault.

Humans have habits because they are efficient; you can perform useful behaviors without wasting time and energy deliberating on what to do. This quick-and-efficient response tendency also has its downsides, especially when bad habits hijack it. Aren't procrastination, telling lies, and deceit also habits?

Habit Formation

The neuroscience

Recent advancements in neuroscience show that our brains are more malleable than we thought. While looking into neuroplasticity, researchers discovered how the connectivity between neurons can change with experience. With practice, these neural networks can form new connections, strengthen existing ones and insulate them, speeding up impulse transmission. We can increase the growth of these neural connections with the actions we take. But I'm getting ahead of myself here. What do neurons have to do with habits?

MIT researchers identified that if neurons fire at the beginning of specific behavior, it becomes a habit. They fire at the start of new behavior and subside after it occurs, then fire again once it's finished. Over time, patterns in the brain known as neural pathways and behavior form and become automatic. That's why breaking a habit is so difficult; it is literally hardwired in your brain.

To better understand how habits are formed, let's look at what goes on in the brain. In the forebrain specifically, an area known as the basal ganglia controls voluntary movement. It also plays a crucial role in the formation of habits—whether good or bad—as well as emotional expression. It helps us form habits so they become automatic, freeing up space in our conscious brain to take on day-to-day activities. These automatic habits include brushing your teeth or driving, and even breathing. However, this area is also responsible for forming unwanted or unhealthy habits such as anxiety, addictions, eating disorders, and so on. Remember, your subconscious mind has no moral compass. It forms habits—both good and bad.

A habit can be described as an instinctive response to a specific situation, acquired from learning and repetition. It is a simplistic form of learning or a behavioral change caused by experience. When a behavior develops to a certain point, it becomes highly automatic and doesn't require conscious attention—it's a habit. Many dominant problems we have in life are preventable. Take, for instance, heart disease. Adopting health-promoting behaviors, such as eating healthier or working out, can significantly improve one's quality of life, both mentally and physically and reduce the chances of getting heart disease. Why not do the same with happiness?

Many times habits are mistaken for routines, with the terms often used interchangeably. While both involve repeated behavior, a routine is not necessarily carried out in response to a desire or craving, like a habit is. You routinely wash the dishes or work out without feeling a desire to do so because you feel you have to do it, with or without a reward. Habits are behaviors that require no conscious thought, while routines require a high degree of intentionality and effort.

People develop habits in the course of pursuing various goals by associating certain cues with behavioral responses that help them meet a goal or obtain a reward. While driving to a certain place, say the beach, you follow particular routes and road markers to get there. Over time, thoughts of the behavior and the behavior itself are triggered by these cues. The same can be said about happiness. When you repeatedly do and spend time thinking about being happy, you will give yourself cues that will trigger future happiness.

Habits are formed physiologically and psychologically. When an act is repeated, various neurons are connected, and a neural pathway is formed. From a psychological standpoint, when a stimulus is related and a specific response is elicited, the connection between them is strengthened, eventually bringing on learning. Psychologically, habits are acquired dispositions born from any learning experience, repeated until it is firmly retained.

The habit loop, a term coined by Charles Duhigg in *The Power of Habit*, describes the various elements that produce habits. These elements are cue, behavior, and reward. Think of them as the steps or backbone of habit formation; your brain goes through them in the same order each time. Breaking down habits to their fundamental parts can help you understand what they are, how they work, and how to change them.

Step 1: The Cue

The cue consists of two parts: the trigger and the craving. The trigger initiates a specific behavior in your brain. It's the information that predicts a reward. Take smokers, for instance—their trigger is usually stress. Whenever they feel anxious, that's their cue to smoke a cigarette. We use a lot of our time learning cues that foretell subsequent rewards such as money, power, fame, status, approval, love, praise, friendship, or personal satisfaction. Your mind is continually on the lookout for external and internal cues of where rewards are located.

Since it is the first indication that you are close to a reward, the cue naturally leads to a craving. Cravings can be thought of as the second part of the cue step. They are the motivating force behind every habit. In our smoker example, the relief a smoker feels, whether physiologically or psychologically, leads to the craving for that relief. This becomes their motivation and desire. Devoid of some motivation or desire, you have no reason to act.

Let's be clear, what you crave is not the habit itself but the change of state it brings. You don't crave junk food—you crave the feeling that eating it brings, that delicious satisfaction of biting into a juicy burger. You don't crave smoking; you are after the relief it provides. You don't actually want to brush your teeth; you want that feeling of fresh breath and a clean mouth. You don't want to watch TV; you want the entertainment it brings. You get the idea? Every craving is attached to a desire to transform your internal state.

Cravings are different for each one of us. Theoretically, anything can trigger a craving; but we are not all motivated by the same cues. For an avid gambler, a slot machines' whirring and chimes are a powerful trigger that ignites an intense desire to play. However, for those who rarely gamble, they are just background noises. Until they are interpreted, triggers are meaningless; it's the thoughts, feelings, and emotions that you attach to them when you sense them that transform them into cravings.

Step 2: The Response or Behavior

The response or behavior is the actual habit you form in response to the cues. It can either be a thought or an action. Whether a behavior occurs will depend on how motivated you are and the work or effort linked with it. If a particular response requires more physical or mental work than you are willing to do, guess what? You won't do it. How you respond to a cue depends on your ability. A habit can only occur if you are capable of it. Take dunking a basketball, for example; if you can't jump high enough, then tough luck, you can't dunk. This doesn't apply to happiness, though; we are all capable of happiness, so you can't use this as an excuse not to be happy.

Step 3: The Reward

Lastly, after the response comes the reward, the end goal of every habit. The trigger is about noticing the reward, the craving is about wanting the reward, and the response is about getting the reward. We chase rewards for two purposes. First, they satisfy our cravings by providing benefits of their own. Food gives you the energy you need. A promotion brings you that feeling you get from getting more money and respect. Working out gets you in shape, improving your health and your dating life. However, a more immediate perk of rewards satisfies your craving to win, improves your status, or fulfills your desire to eat. Rewards temporarily deliver contentment and relief from our cravings.

Secondly, rewards teach us the actions worth remembering. Since your brain is a reward detector, it constantly monitors which actions satisfy your desires and please you as you go about your day. Pleasure and frustration are part of the feedback mechanism that helps the brain discern useful and useless actions. Rewards are the last step in the habit loop; they close the habit cycle.

If any behavior falls short during any of these steps, it doesn't become a habit. If you take out the cue, your habit is never triggered. Reduce the craving, and you lack the motivation to do it. Make the behavior difficult and you won't have the ability to do it. If the reward fails to satisfy your craving, there's no reason to repeat it. What I want you to understand is that a habit needs all three steps to form. Without all three, the behavior won't occur or be repeated.

These stages of habit formation create an endless cycle that runs every minute of every day. This system constantly searches the environment, trying to predict what will happen, trying out different responses, and learning from the results. The cue activates a craving, which motivates an action that yields a reward that gratifies the said craving, which now becomes associated with the triggering cue. Together, they form a neurological loop, cue-craving-response-reward, which ultimately creates automatic habits. This means they form neural pathways in this pattern for every behavior.

Habit formation can more simply be split into two phases—the problem and the solution. The problem phase includes the trigger and craving, when you realize something needs to change. The solution phase includes the response and reward, where you take action to achieve your desired goal. Understand that all behavior is driven by a desire to solve a problem and habits are how you do this. You wake up, you want to feel more alert, so you drink a cup of coffee. Drinking coffee satisfies your craving to be alert, so it becomes associated with waking up.

When you are grown up, you barely notice the habits running your life. You never give another thought to how you always change into more comfortable clothes after getting home. Decades of mental programming eventually turn into automatic thought patterns and actions.

THREE

How to Build Better Habits in Simple Steps

OLD HABITS ARE a pain to shake off, and developing new ones is even harder. However, it is possible. So how do you create new habits? Well, we have already gone through step one, understanding how habits are formed. By understanding how a habit is formed, you are gaining insight into your habits and yourself. You have a better chance when you know what you are up against. This is a war, a war for your happiness, and right now, the bad habits keeping you from living a happier life are winning.

Why It's So Hard to Change

There is a lot of information and advice on how to change your life for the better and when you go through it, sometimes you think, "no way, I can't do that." Other times you think, "this is definitely for me." However, whenever you try to implement the advice, the change only lasts for a short time, and then you are back to your old habits. So, why is it so hard to change your behavior, thoughts, and habits?

Take a moment and cross your legs. Now, cross them in the opposite direction. Which way felt more awkward to you? If you think that it was the second one because it required some thought, then you are right. When you crossed your legs the first time, the signal came from a different part of your mind than it did the next time around. Habits are the choices we make deliberately up to a point when they become automatic.

That is why you didn't have to think about which way to cross your legs the first time. Habits make up more than 40 percent of what we do every day because the brain is lazy in a way; it doesn't want to have to think about every little thing you do all the time, so it forms habits. The only problem is it can't tell the difference between good and bad habits. It takes everything you say, do, and think repeatedly and turns it into a habit, so it doesn't have to think so hard all the time.

When you crossed your legs the first time, the signals came from your subconscious mind. The second time, the signals came from your conscious mind because you were actively thinking about crossing your legs in the opposite direction. Your first actions were basically on autopilot, and you didn't have to do any thinking.

If you hate your job or are dreading going to work, your mind will immediately go into a negative mindset, which then triggers the preset emotions and actions you are used to. You end up starting your day the same way you always have, in a grumpy, bad mood, and as such, all your actions will seem only to worsen your mood. It might seem like the world is conspiring against you, but in essence, this is all on you.

Your past, present, and future become predictable because you are operating from the same habit (thought-feeling) pattern. If you are used to quitting a job after three months, you will find that whenever you get a new position, you always find a way to quit or sabotage yourself after three months or around that time. If you are an emotional eater, someone who uses food to bury their feelings, you might find that no matter what you do, you are unable to change that because your body and your emotions are addicted to it. This is also why people find it hard to quit smoking, lose weight, get a steady job, and be in a stable relationship.

We resist change because it messes with our natural habits and thought-feeling patterns. Whether it is a new role, job, diet, or routine, your brain has to work to learn how to adapt to the changes. When you start changing, your body protests because what you are feeling is not the way you are used to. Your brain doesn't know what is happening, and it doesn't like the fact that it has to work so hard now. Why does the conscious mind think it can just wake up, start thinking, and take over things again? The current blueprint works just fine, so why would you change it? And thus begins the fight between your conscious and subconscious mind, as they battle it out for control, and if you are not careful, you will fall back onto your old habits and thought-emotion pattern addictions.

Let's take losing weight, for instance. You wake up one day, try putting on your favorite outfit, and it doesn't fit. You look in the mirror and you are shocked at how much your body has changed. You then decide that you are going to lose weight. You find a good gym and even pay for a membership, buy workout clothes, and go for the first three sessions with a lot of excitement. But on the fourth day, this high is over; you wake up feeling lazy, sore, and you feel like every single muscle is aching. At that moment, you might ask yourself whether it is really worth it or would it be easier to quit. All these aches and pains are the body's way of trying to get you to quit so you can go back to what it's already used to.

Others don't even make it to the gym. The thought of starting a workout routine is marred by thoughts such as, "But I work until late, when will I have time to work out? I'm so fat, what will people think of me when I go to the gym?" Eventually, these thoughts weigh them down, and they never even get started.

How to Change Your Habits

Changing old habits requires that you change your thoughts and emotions and form new habits, a process that can be very uncomfortable. The more ingrained these thoughts and habits are, the harder and longer it takes to change and form new ones. That is why the things we go through as children and the habits we form from these experiences stay with us well into adulthood. An example is thinking that you are not worthy because you were raised by a narcissistic parent. However, it is not all bad; you can change even the most ingrained thought patterns and habits if you intentionally train your mind to think and behave in new ways. Plus, the more you do it, the more natural it becomes to form new habits.

Remember the steps of habit formation? Well, we can turn it into practical frameworks that you can use to change your habits and even eliminate bad ones. Think of each stage as a building block that influences your behavior. If you use them correctly, you'll be able to change habits. To create a new habit, make the cue obvious, the craving attractive, the response easy, and the reward satisfying.

Given the cue-dependent automatic nature of habits, channeling these fundamental laws of habit formation is the key to creating new habits. Adding the habit formation components to any attempt at real behavioral change can help shield your new habits from motivational lapses and increase the chance of them lasting long-term. For some behavior, one instance is enough to attain the desired result. For example, taking a single vacation can help you relax faster and drastically reduce your stress levels. However, for most behavior, repetitive action is required to achieve meaningful outcomes. To achieve long-term happiness, for instance, you have to deliberately cultivate a culture of gratitude and service. In such instances, habit change must be viewed as a long-term process divided into two steps —initiation and maintenance.

This distinction is important because many people fail at attaining long-term change despite having the capability, opportunity, and motivation to initiate the change. They often go back to old habits after a drop in motivation. New Year's resolutions, anyone? This change can be attributed to a drop in motivation after the initial experiences of the new habit.

People can also overestimate the positive outcomes of the actions they take to change and feel disappointed when the outcomes fall short of their expectations or fail to factor in negative outcomes. Alternatively, a newly acquired habit can lose its value and become deprioritized over time. What I'm trying to say is that a loss in motivation can permanently derail any successful attempts of behavioral change.

So, to change, you need to overwrite your thought and emotion blueprint and kill the bad habit. This is the only way to show your subconscious mind and your body that the conscious mind is in control. You start by noticing or becoming aware of your thought patterns (cues) and the results of these patterns. You also need to become aware of your thought tone; is it positive or negative? In this case, it is negative, so make the conscious decision to change. Remember, your subconscious mind will try to distract you from your new path, so you'll have to stay strong.

Let's say you are an emotional eater. Every time you feel the urge to eat, be mindful of your thoughts and feelings at that time. Do this every time you get these urges and take note of the most common emotions, thoughts, and factors that lead to these urges. This is the realization step; you realize that you have a problem and what thoughts or feelings cause it. It's better than denying the truth that you have a problem because suppressed emotions only feed the subconscious mind the same negative emotional patterns that you are trying to change or eliminate.

There are several things you can do to help you change your mindset. You can set goals, so you have something to focus on, using positive affirmations or the power of repetition and meditation to change how you think and feel. Meditation is the best way to clear negative beliefs from your mind and life while fostering emotional and spiritual healing. It renews the mind and body and calms your inner being. Through meditation, you can rewire your brain and tune it into positive thinking vibes.

Since habits form from what you do rather than what you think, here are some simple hacks to help you create good habits:

Define your context—context here refers to your immediate environment, except yourself. This includes where you live, the people you are with, what time of day it is, and even the actions you perform.

Just as you would gather your ingredients so it's easier to cook, you need to organize your environment to make it easier for you to do the same thing repeatedly. We don't often realize how much our environment and the pressures around us drive our actions. If you want to stop binge eating, remove the temptation. That is the food. Eat tiny healthy portions more frequently during the day so that you are not starving by the time you get to your main meal.

Repeat, repeat, repeat—a behavior will only turn into a habit through conscious repetition. This consistency increases its accessibility and prominence, so when you are in a similar context, the habit automatically kicks in. Logically, you may be wondering just how long it takes to build a habit. Well, popular opinion says it only takes 21 days to create a habit, but studies have proven that it takes anywhere between 6 to 9 months to effectively build a habit. With the increased timeline, you run the risk of losing momentum and motivation along the way, as well as finding the habit less rewarding. However, don't you think that forming a new habit of self-love is worth it?

Up the rewards—with an organized context and repetition to jumpstart your habit building, you need to sweeten the deal if you are to actually succeed and get these habits to operate on their own. The rewards have to be bigger and better than what you would normally expect. When it comes to behavioral change, intrinsic motivation, the internal force that pushes you, is invaluable. However, incentives come in really handy at this point. They can help with habit building by motivating you even more to engage in the desired behavior.

This is because unexpected rewards spur the release of dopamine, a feel-good hormone, that etches the circumstances of the rewarding experience into memory, making you more likely to repeat the behavior. This creates an energy that invigorates you to pursue actions that have positive outcomes and achieve your happiness goals. If you want to work out because it boosts your moods but you hate going to the gym, you are not going to get in shape unless you add something, such as listening to music while working out, to entice you into doing it. The more fun it is, the more likely you are to turn it into a habit.

If you still have trouble building healthy habits, you can try:

- **Stacking**—rather than making a big change at once, start small. Try forming a habit by taking advantage of an existing behavior to cue a new one in. For instance, if you have some medication to take after breakfast, placing it on the table when you eat (morning habit) automatically reminds you to take it after breakfast. To build long-term self-love habits, try stacking them onto other habits. As you learn to forgive yourself for mistakes, you are working on being kinder to yourself.
- **Swapping**—it pretty much means exactly that; swap out a habit you already have with something similar. If you want to stop drinking soda, try switching to bottled tea. Since the packaging is the same, and you carry and use it just like a soda, the substitution will be easier to accept. Rather than looking to others for ideas, look inwards.

There are a couple of things to keep in mind when navigating change.

1. You cannot use logic to counter your emotions. Change can be scary, and we often feel anxiety, insecurities, and fear of the unknown. Even though the change might be logical, such as losing weight due to health reasons, knowing this does nothing to alleviate the feelings of discomfort associated with it. You have to give yourself time to process the emotions you are feeling instead of suppressing or trying to ignore them. Realize why you feel this way, and don't be judgmental about your feelings.

Just acknowledge that you have these feelings and observe them. Don't try to take on your goals while going through these emotions. Stop, observe, acknowledge, feel them, and then move on to the next step.

2. Understand what you are getting out of this. Even if the change is for your own good, it is easier to resist it and keep your old habits. Take some time to ask yourself and identify what's in it for me? This will be your motivator through the discomfort.

If you cannot find a positive reason why you should do this, think of the negative result you want to avoid.

3. Identify any hurdles you might face and how to handle them. It is about managing the negative self-talk that might affect you as you try to achieve your goals. If you want to healthily shed some weight, you will have to exercise more and change your diet and eating habits. And while weight loss can help you get healthier, factors such as time, money, lifestyle, or laziness can interfere. So, as you set your weight loss goals, also make plans on how to deal with these barriers.

For instance, plan your meals so that you always have healthy food options no matter where you go. If you are too tired to work out after work, try sleeping in your workout clothes and wake up earlier to get that workout in.

4. Surround yourself with the right people. Changing your habits is hard enough without having people around you telling you that you will fail or to just give up.

These energy drainers can cause you to quit or deviate from your goals, so surround yourself with those who support you instead.

5. Think about the big picture. Change can be daunting, but once you are through to the other side, you can look back and see your growth.

Shifting your mindset is the first step, and keeping the bigger picture in mind can help keep you motivated through the pain and challenges you will face.

6. If you want to behave differently, then think differently. When you change your mindset, the results will show up accordingly. You can retrain your mind and form new thoughts, patterns, and habits with a little courage and readiness to go out of your comfort zone. The process can be scary, but by managing it, you can set yourself up for success.

How to Increase Your Self-Control

On your journey to better yourself, love yourself more, and change your bad habits, you need more than good intentions to get things done. After looking at how habits and behaviors are formed, you understand how hard it is to change. Sticking to one plan is pretty hard, and humans are notoriously poor at following through, even when they know it's for the best. We tend to be very indecisive about change and somewhat resistant to it. Take, for instance, losing weight; even though you know you need to lose weight, you still eat junk food. This is because these behaviors and habits are already ingrained in our subconscious, and changing them means actively engaging the conscious mind, which is tiring.

Defining Self-Control

Self-control, willpower, and self-discipline all describe the same thing—the ability or effort to regulate potentially bad responses in service of a higher goal. This choice, however, is not automatic but rather a conscious decision you make. The American Psychological Association (APA) gives these characteristics of self-control:

- The ability to stop an impulsive response that could potentially undo your commitment.
- The capability to postpone gratification, countering short-term temptations to meet long-term goals.
- The capacity to be cool rather than hot-headed, emotionally.

To initiate and sustain the change, you need self-control. Understand that you are going against behaviors you have had for a long time. You need something extra to propel and sustain the new habits. However, self-control isn't a character strength most people naturally have. This ability to control your feelings, reactions, and emotions is crucial in the world we live in. After all, we have to deal with stress, change, and challenges at every turn, so being able to calmly navigate these situations is vital.

Aside from this, self-control is a crucial component of leading a more successful and satisfying life. However, self-control is a limited resource that gets depleted with use. This means that if you were to exercise self-control in one situation, there's a high chance you will lose it in the next one. Self-control is an act of willpower, meaning the more you use it, the less of it you have, which leads you to eventually lose your self-control. Luckily there are several ways you can lessen this willpower depletion and even enhance your self-control.

Look at the big picture

A simple way to detach yourself and prevent things from overwhelming you is by looking at the bigger picture. A study on self-control shows that abstract or higher-level thinking increases your success of gaining self-control. This study explains that our mental representations of events heavily impact our self-control. It also proposes that you are more likely to exercise self-control if you focus on the proverbial forest that lies beyond the one tree currently blocking your view. For instance, if you're working on a year-long project, it's easy for you to get sidetracked and frustrated by the many challenges you face along the way. However, suppose you periodically remind yourself to look at the forest rather than the trees. In that case, you can focus on the end game—completing the project rather than getting discouraged along the way.

Develop self-awareness

This basically means to know thyself. How many temptations can you resist in a day? One or twenty? Maybe more than twenty? It's impossible to know because we make most of our decisions unconsciously. However, by becoming more self-aware by getting more attuned to when, where, and how you exercise self-control, you can manage your behavior a lot better. For example, if you were to go to the supermarket on an empty stomach, there's a high chance that you'd make several impulse buys, most of which you wouldn't have made had you gone on a full stomach. If you are aware of this, you know that you should probably eat first before going shopping. This way you don't spend money on food that you would have spent on something else. Gaining self-awareness is the first step to making better decisions and resisting those that don't help long term. By knowing yourself better, you can recognize and avoid temptation either by avoiding it or by distracting yourself.

On that note, you want to avoid decision fatigue. If you make too many decisions, no matter how small, you will quickly use up your willpower and compromise your self-control. Decision fatigue adversely impacts your decisions, and in some cases, you might find that you prefer not making a choice at all or you become impulsive. Take judges, for instance; they are known to make poorer decisions at the end of the day because they are tired. You need to preserve your decision-making energy, and a great way to do this is routinizing yourself. This way, you don't get distracted by trivial decisions.

Get enough sleep

I can't stress this enough; you have to get enough quality sleep. A research study done by the University of Washington showed that sleep deprivation drains glucose levels in the prefrontal cortex, therefore depleting your fuel for willpower. When you get quality sleep, you can restore these glucose levels. The study found that getting enough quality sleep makes a great difference the next day, especially when choosing between ethical and unethical behavior. People who sleep for about 6 hours or less are more likely to engage in aggressive behavior than those who sleep for 7 to 9 hours.

Exercise and relax

Exercise can be defined as any movement that moves your muscles and burns calories. It includes physical activities such as swimming, running, jogging, and dancing. There are many benefits to exercising, such as boosting happiness levels, easing anxiety and stress, increasing energy levels, boosting your brain health and memory, and helping with relaxation and sleep. To enhance your self-control, you need enough rest and sleep to recharge, and working out can help with that. Working out increases your blood and oxygen flow to the prefrontal cortex, meaning you can boost your self-control ability.

That said, you have to take some time off to kick back and relax.

Taking a pause every once in a while can help you be less impulsive; this relaxed state allows you to have more control over your temptations, automatically kicking in your self-control. If you don't get enough rest, you are probably going to be cranky and not want to have to think about making decisions. Relaxing doesn't have to mean taking a 2-week holiday on a warm sunny beach; even taking a few seconds to rev down can make a huge difference.

Lastly, understand that self-control is not about deprivation or punishment. It is about redefining what you find pleasurable to help keep destructive behaviors in check. It's about having power over your actions and learning how to ignore impulses no matter how strong they are.

How to make your habits engaging—Make big goals and small quotas

Your motivation to change is tied to the goals you make and the habits you want to form to achieve these goals. A study done on motivation showed that abstract thinking is a great way of helping with discipline. You know that popular saying "dream big." Turns out it's pretty good advice after all. That said, we often have trouble coming up with grand plans because we end up being intimidated by our own lofty goals. You could decide that you want to start your own business in two years but then chicken out when you actually think of everything that starting a business entails.

Researchers have found that creating intrinsic motivators is an essential part of making new habits stick. Your dream is not far-fetched: you just have to split it up into smaller, more easily achievable quotas. Your goals represent the big picture you want to achieve, while your quotas are the bare minimums you have to do to achieve these goals.

For instance, if you want to be a writer, writing about 1000 words a day will help improve your writing skills and push you to achieve your dreams. Let's say you are trying to floss more. You can commit yourself to floss one tooth every time you brush your teeth. You could decide to floss all of them, but the daily quota to meet is flossing one tooth. Ever so often, you might floss just one tooth, but most of the time, you will floss them all. This simple technique works really well when trying to learn new behaviors.

The Role of Those Close to You in Shaping Your Habits

When working on changing your habits, you have to understand that your environment plays a big role in shaping your behavior. Your environment encompasses more than just where you live, work or hang out; it includes the people you interact with in these places— your family and friends. Most people think that self-control and willpower only come from within; however, most of your actions depend on your friends and family as much as yourself.

The people around you have the power to influence what you think, feel, and do. For instance, they can make you eat healthily or choose junk food. This is not merely peer pressure where you deliberately act in a certain way to fit into a group. The effect family and friends have on your behavior is largely unconscious. Your subconscious mind is constantly picking up cues from these people, which in turn informs your behavior. While it may not look like a big deal, the consequences can be serious.

Our sense of self is derived from other people; we tend to draw our identity from the group of people we associate with the most. Even when you are not with them, you still exhibit the values, habits, and thought patterns you got from the group. The more you interact with someone, the greater their influence on you. While our minds influence our actions, the people around us tend to be our greatest influencers.

This influencing power can be classified under nature or nurture. Your nature is the preference you are born with, while nurture covers how you are shaped by those closest to you and the environment you are in. Nature gives way to nurture as we begin to mature and interact with others. Family members often have a strong, nurturing influence on us because they are the people we socialize with first. Additionally, because we are attracted to people with whom we share commonalities, we are open to being influenced by our peers.

For example, if you take part in a sport, you might consider your teammates to be your peers. However, just because you play the same sport, you might not have other shared interests. That's why it's so hard to look at family and friends' influences independently of each other. We work very close to them and the initial influence family has on us can affect who we become in the future. During adolescence, most kids experiment with finding their own identities, and sometimes it ends up being the absolute opposite of what their parents want.

As you can see, those around us have a strong influence on us; however, this is a double-edged sword. In the face of criticism from a stranger, you will come to the aid of your friend; however, if you are left to form your own opinions, you might interpret hypocritical behavior as a sign to relax your views. This behavior is referred to as vicarious dissonance. It's when you see someone behaving in a way that's inconsistent with your own values and attitudes. This makes you likely to change them.

For example, the way we talk about our health choices with those close to us can significantly impact our decisions. If they are not as accepting of your ideas, they might cause you not to follow through with the changes. Anything those close to us do or say can influence us, whether we are conscious of it or not. Their support can decide whether you act in the right way or not. The presence of others clouds our ability to pick up on the cues our bodies are sending. For instance, the feeling of being full is often disrupted in the presence of your friends, which results in you eating more.

The influence family and friends have on us can be referred to as social norms. If you are with a new social group, you are more likely to adopt their social norms. If you hang out with people who like drinking, you will start drinking to fit in. Your decisions might not always be up to you because you are susceptible to the influence of others. This doesn't have to be a bad thing, though. Bad influence is as easy to spread as good influence. Remember that.

FOUR

How a Responsible Partner Gives You a Different Perspective in Life and Helps You Find Happiness

WHILE WE MUST FIND happiness within ourselves, this doesn't mean ignoring the people around us. We often have very negative, unintentional relationships with those around us, even when they can seem quite positive in the beginning. When we get into relationships, we get trapped into trying to take on a lot of the other people's problems and trying to get them to fix our problems in turn. This can create a psychological image of who we think they are and, in turn, who they think we are. However, this psychological image or the expectations we set are quite far from reality, which only complicates our interpersonal relationships.

It may seem odd to look at relationships after having spoken so much about ourselves and how we are solely responsible for our happiness. However, a large body of research and psychological studies highlight the importance of good, healthy relationships. They help us to learn, grow, laugh, and love. Those with robust, broad-ranging social connections are happier, flourishing, and tend to live longer. Good relationships with loved ones, relatives and friends provide love, meaning, comfort and raise our sense of self-worth. Widening our social networks brings a sense of belonging, so strengthening our kinships and building quality connections is integral to finding true happiness.

Relationships are the backbone of a meaningful life. When surrounded by others, we tend to define ourselves by our relationships. Humans are not solitary creatures; from birth, we depend on others for survival, both physically and spiritually. Life is better when we share our wins and losses with others. The quality of the relationships we have largely determines the quality of life we have. If you have loving, supporting relationships, you are generally happier and more open to others. You are easy-going and can take on challenges because you know someone has your back. Your quality of life is good.

The reverse also holds. Devoid of love and support, we feel something is lacking in our lives. Even though happiness comes from within, it is generated by the interactions between our thoughts and the state of our bodies. However, external factors, such as lack of love, support, and loneliness, can heavily influence our internal state. It stands to reason that our external environment affects our internal landscape. If you are struggling to find happiness within, changing your external landscape by building good relationships can declutter your internal environment. By purging the things that don't do us any good or bring us joy, we are left with what does. Building good relationships allows us to bring those positive things into view and serves as an example of how to declutter and change our internal state.

Why Relationships Matter

Relationships contribute to overall happiness and wellbeing. It's about social connectedness and having love and intimacy in your life through friends, family, and romantic partners. Wellbeing and happiness drawn from good relationships are characterized by the fact that by caring for others and in turn being cared for, both needs are satisfied. When two people put the other's wellbeing ahead of themselves then both can be happy. When it comes to social connections, most of us are winging it. We are often swept off our feet and exhilarated by the early stages of love, but the grind of daily life and our personal baggage start to creep in after a while. We find ourselves struggling in the face of hurt, emotional withdrawal, worsening conflict, boredom, and inadequate coping mechanisms. We soon realize that building happy and healthy relationships is hard. It takes work.

There's a lot of research on relationships, with scientists trying to figure out what the healthiest and happiest couples are doing right. Harvard currently has the longest ongoing study of relationships in human history. The study aims to answer the question of what makes life good. In the 1930s, Harvard researchers invited several sophomores from the school and teenagers from some of Boston's poorest neighborhoods to participate in a study. They were 19 at the time. Over the next 75 years, they were interviewed, had medical tests done, and were checked up on every two years to see how they were doing. What the researchers found out about happiness surprised them.

Many people think that fame, fortune, and hard work will bring them happiness; however, they don't. It's the social connections we have that are most vital to our happiness and wellbeing. But how can someone who worked so hard to earn fame and fortune be unhappy? The Harvard researchers learned three key lessons. First, good relationships are good for our bodily health and wellbeing, and loneliness and being separated from others can literally kill. Secondly, it's the quality, not the quantity of relationships that matters. Lastly, good relationships are not only good for your body but also your mind.

What the longest study on happiness teaches us

Sting was at the height of his music career in 1983. The Police, his band, had topped the charts with their recent album, and their song was the most played song on the radio. Albums were flying off the shelves and concerts were selling out. It appeared like all was going according to plan. Sting and The Police had a successful music career and all the fame and money they could want. However, they broke up the following year. Why?

The answer is quite simple; pop culture had the wrong idea of happiness because there's a disconnect between what we think, imagine, or believe will make us happy versus what actually does. That's why people think that fame and fortune are the keys to happiness. Pop culture drummed this idea into their minds through images and videos. However, this has nothing to do with finding happiness. The world is littered with unhappy rich people, tormented celebrities, and lonely workaholics.

What makes us truly happy are the good relationships we have. The Harvard researchers found that making social connections is good for your physical health. Those connected to family, friends, and community were happier, physically healthier, and lived longer. Loneliness has a deeply detrimental effect on people. The study proved it. Those who were segregated from others or had fewer social connections were often lonely. Loneliness increases the chances of getting a heart attack by over 40 percent. Your risk of premature death grows by over 50 percent.

The scientists also determined that it's not the number of connections or relationships you have but the quality that matters. Those who valued quantity over quality had poorer physical health and were less happy than those who had fewer but better relationships. Focusing on quantity reduces the quality of the connections you make, while reducing the number of relationships you have allows you to focus on their quality. High-quality relationships are resonant, while low-quality ones are dissonant. This means that high-quality relationships are characterized by mutual trust and respect, while low-quality ones are more conflict-prone. The distinction between the two is due to the different neurological networks that form and trigger when we connect with others. Resonant relationships trigger connections in parts of the brain associated with positive emotion. In contrast, dissonant relationships trigger parts of the brain linked to avoidance, decreased compassion and affection, and other negative emotions.

Our brains remember and react to the quality of the connections we make. The quality of these relationships has long influenced various aspects of our physical and psychological health. Ask yourself, are your personal relationships bringing out the best in you? Do they make you a better person? Do you find yourself uplifted whenever you are around your family or friends?

Having high-quality relationships also benefits the mind. The study showed that those with better social relationships had sharper memory, while those in poorer relationships showed a sharp decline in memory. These relationships reduce the risk of getting dementia and other mental decline conditions. Forming quality social connections has been proven to lower anxiety and depression and boost self-esteem, empathy, trust, and cooperation. They also reduce stress, which boosts your immune system too.

The great thing about building good relationships is that they make you happier and more satisfied with life. They protect you from life's stresses and also trigger a flow-on effect, where those surrounding you will be drawn into spending more time with you because you are literally a "ray of sunshine." In this way, social connectedness creates a positive feedback loop of social, physical, and emotional wellbeing. People will naturally be attracted to knowing you and being with you.

How Your Mindset Can Affect Your Relationships

People with a fixed mindset feel threatened and are often hostile when talking about even minor issues about how they or their significant other see their relationship. They believe that they are one with their partner and share the same views, so even a minor disagreement can threaten this belief. The most cataclysmic of all relationship myths that those with a fixed mindset have is the belief that if it requires work, then something is very wrong and that even the slightest difference in opinion or choice is a sign of a character flaw in their partners. However, by now, you know better. There are no great accomplishments without setbacks, so there are no great relationships without disagreements and issues along the way.

If you have a fixed mindset whenever you talk about the conflicts in your relationship, you tend to place blame. It could be on yourself, but a lot of the time, it's your partner's fault. This blame is assigned to a trait or a character flaw. As if that's not enough, this blame game causes you to feel anger and disdain toward your partner. And it gets worse; since the issue stems from permanent traits, it can't be solved. Once you see them in your partner, you become scornful and condescending to them and unhappy with the whole relationship.

However, with a growth mindset, you can acknowledge your partner's flaws without placing blame, and still feel that you have a fulfilling connection. You view conflicts as indicators of communication issues, not as a sign of issues with your personality. This holds true both in intimate partnerships, friendships, and also in your relationship with your parents.

When we set out to build a relationship, we meet someone totally different from us, and we don't know how to handle these differences yet. In a working relationship, we build these skills by spending time together, showing interest in each other, and emotionally nurturing one another. This grows and deepens the relationship. However, for this to occur, we've got to be on the same page or at least feel like we are. As trust develops, we become interested in each other's progress. When we form bonds, we tend to adapt to them, often getting complacent in the long run. We take how things are a reality rather than working on them to make our relationships work. Understand you cannot have a perfect relationship; aim for a 5:1 ratio of positive to negative feelings. After all, it's the negative emotions that provide hidden opportunities to learn more about each other.

What all your interactions culminate in is your mindset. This is an explanatory process that explains what's going on around you. The fixed mindset is marred by an intrinsic monologue of continuous judging and analysis, using all the information you observe as proof either for or against assessments such as whether you or someone else is inherently good. Does he or she have the traits to be a good match for you, or are you better than them? The internal monologue of the growth mindset is not as judgmental, but it is eager to learn and hungry for information. This mindset is constantly on the lookout for the kind of input you can absorb into learning and helpful action.

Building Healthy Relationships

Many of our kinships are formed accidentally. You probably met your friends or spouse at work, at school, at a club, or while randomly walking down the street. It happens. It's safe to say that the relationships you have in your life right now are based on proximity. This is because it is simple and convenient for us to form connections with those we are around most of the time. There's nothing wrong with it, except we aren't intentional about it. We leave this important decision up to a random choice such as where we live, where we work, or where we go to school.

These relationships are formed because they are effortless and comfortable; however, they may not always be ideal for us. "Show me your mates, and I will tell you the type of person you are" is a saying that sums it up quite nicely. Given that we are not intentional about the relationships we form, we leave ourselves open to opportunistic and toxic relationships and social connections.

Look at the connections in your life right now and ask yourself:

- Does it make me feel good?
- Does it offer as much or more than it takes? Conversely, do I give more into it than what I take?
- Does it serve me and the other person and does it bring us both joy?

I figure there are several people and relationships that would answer some or all these questions with a hard no. For these people, I would like to ask why are you still hanging on? If a relationship doesn't make sense, keeping it won't change that; dropping it may even make you happier. Decluttering your closet and donating some of your old clothes can make you happy; you will feel that you have done some good. The same goes for relationships. Dropping those relationships that no longer make us happy is like decluttering your life. Many of the relationships we have, we maintain them because they are easy, and we want to avoid the emotional effort required to let go. Remember, we are averse to loss, so our minds would rather stay with a failed relationship than deal with the emotional fallout that marks the end of it.

Just like that pair of jeans that don't fit anymore, these relationships had a point but now they have run their course. They probably made us happy once, so we keep them because of what they represent and because we are too lazy or nostalgic to end them, even though, deep down, we know that they will no longer make us happy. To be truly happy, we have to let go of the emotional clutter, unhealthy attachments, and connections that take more than they give. It's the essence of living a happier life. Removing the negative is just as important as adding the good stuff, and nowhere does it have a more significant impact than on our relationships.

It might seem harsh talking about your relationships with such ruthless precision; however, it's for the best. The only connections worth building are where both parties benefit from them.

There are three types of social connections you can have:

Intimate—such as those between you and the people you love and care for—your family, friends, and lovers.

Relational—these are formed with the people you see often and have a shared interest, such as your workmates or business friends.

Collective—these connections are formed between people who share a group membership or affiliation, such as the people you go to church or the gym with and people who share your political views.

When building relationships, ask yourself, do you have good, meaningful, long-term relationships in these areas? Maybe you tend to stick with old friends and feel you can't meet new people? Or maybe you are avoiding people from your past and mingling with people who know as little about you as possible? Be honest about your relationships and social connections. Think about the relationships you have had and the type of relationships you would like to have. You may find that you would want to try making new friends despite sticking with old ones for so long, or you may want to strengthen existing relationships.

A simple way to bolster existing social connections is to reach out to people you already know, such as family, friends, neighbors, or coworkers with whom you want to build a good relationship. Give them a call. Write or message them on social media; let them know you'd like to keep in touch more. Plan coffee dates, picnics, go swimming, or play a round of golf together. Think about common interests you share and use that to find things to do together.

To meet new people, you can strike up a conversation with someone you regularly see on the train, the bus, at the gym, or even at your favorite coffee place. You can join a team or volunteer. Engaging in community service is a great way to build social connections. Find out about local groups or programs by visiting your local community center or public library; there's always something happening in your community.

Having these fun times will help you develop more positive feelings towards people and share in the happiness that comes from engaging positively with others. The idea behind building good relationships is sharing your time and experiences with the people you want and also listening to them. Remember to be intentional about the relationships and social connections you create. Over time, you will create meaningful and intentional relationships with those you care about. These relationships will benefit your mind and body.

That being said, it doesn't mean that you should accept everyone. Remember, be intentional. Relationships are messy, and not every person can be your friend. While you may genuinely want to build a good relationship with someone, it doesn't always work out. Sometimes it's best to end a toxic relationship no matter what stage it is in. This intentionality helps ground us in reality, rather than floating away into the clouds of expectation as we so often do, especially when relationships come into play.

With a clearer view, we can see people for who they are, not who we expect them to be, and we can connect with them better. This allows us to water and nurture the relationships we want in our lives, much like flowers in a garden, so that they grow strong and supportive.

FIVE

How to Deal with Stress

STRESS AFFECTS EVERYBODY, but whenever we hear the word, our minds automatically think of the adverse effects it has. Whether we are at home, at work, thinking about our finances, or some challenges we may be facing, we are constantly under stress; it is everywhere. A little bit of stress is not bad; it can even be beneficial sometimes. However, too much stress is detrimental to your health. Most people don't truly understand what stress is and often figure out that they are stressed when it's already too late, and they are about to break down. So what is stress exactly? Let's have a look.

What Is Stress?

Defining stress is a bit tricky since it's a highly subjective occurrence. As it is widely used today, the term "stress" can be defined as the body's nonspecific reaction to any demands for change. It was coined by Hans Selye, a Hungarian Canadian endocrinologist who researched the hypothetical non-scientific response of organisms to stressors. He stated that stress occurs whether you receive good or bad news or if the impulse is negative or positive.

Hans Selye's research into stress is how we learned about the stress response. This response occurs in 3 phases—the initial alarm phase, followed by a resistance or adaptation phase, and eventually exhaustion and death. The alarm phase refers to the initial symptoms of the body when under stress. This fight-or-flight response makes you either flee or protect yourself in bad situations. In this stage, your heart rate increases, cortisol and adrenaline are released, which increases your energy, and your muscles tense, ready for what might happen. Your immune and digestive systems are slowed down because all your energy is focused on helping you get out of danger.

The second stage, or the resistance phase, comes after the fight or flight response, when the body begins mending itself. Cortisol and adrenaline levels fall, and your pulse rate and blood pressure begin to go back to their normal levels. However, even though your body has entered the recovery phase, it's still on high alert. If you happened to have dealt with what was causing the stress and it is no longer an issue, your body will continue with its repairs, regulating your hormonal levels, blood pressure, and heart rate.

However, if your stress persists, your body will remain in this heightened state of alertness, and it will eventually adapt to living with a higher stress level and undergoes changes you might not be aware of. You will continue secreting cortisol, adrenaline, and other hormones, which will keep your heart rate and blood pressure high. This heightened state of alertness will also make you irritable, frustrated, and unfocused. If you remain in the resistance stage for too long without dealing with your stressors, it can lead to the exhaustion stage.

The last stage comes as a result of prolonged or chronic stress. It occurs when you have struggled with stress for so long that it has drained you physically, mentally, and emotionally, and you no longer have the strength to fight your stress. At this point, you feel helpless, tired, or hopeless. You might also experience fatigue, burnout, depression, anxiety, along with decreased tolerance for existing or new stress (read as little to no willpower). Your immunity at this point is quite weakened because it has been suppressed for quite a while, leaving you prone to opportunistic and stress-related illnesses.

Whenever you feel threatened, whether it's real or not, your body releases chemicals that enable you to protect yourself from injury. These chemicals—cortisol, adrenaline, and noradrenaline—can increase your heart rate, raise your blood pressure, and make you more alert. This stress response or reaction is known as fight-or-flight and is essential for survival. This heightened state fuels you to deal with the threat and improves your ability to handle the dangerous or challenging situation.

Factors that can lead to stress are referred to as stressors, and they can include noise, scary moments, your first day at work, fighting with your spouse, almost hitting a car in traffic, and others. The more stressors you are under, the more stressed you get.

In most people, the stress response can be triggered easily; for instance, when we are subjected to too many stressors at once, such as is the case with everyday life, our stress response kicks in. Ideally, once the threat has passed, your body is supposed to revert to its normal, relaxed state. Unfortunately, due to the continuous, nonstop demands and complications of everyday modern life, there's always something new stressing you out, so your internal alarm systems never shut off.

Stress means different things to everyone. What might be stressing you could be of little concern to someone else. We get stressed when the demands of life become too much, and we struggle to cope with them. These demands vary and can be anything from family to finances, careers, relationships, or any situations that might pose a real or perceived challenge or threat to your wellbeing.

People also handle stress differently—some are able to handle the pressure while others buckle under it. When faced with challenging situations, it is how we react to them that determines how much stress we will be under and the effects it will have on our health. If you feel that you might be lacking the resources needed to resolve your stressful situation, or you might have a stronger reaction to stress, it can eventually have severe outcomes. If, on the other hand, you feel that you have the right resources to handle the situation, your stress levels are more likely to be lower with fewer resultant health problems.

Here's the thing, stress doesn't necessarily have to come from bad experiences. Even positive experiences, such as giving birth to a baby, taking a trip with your family, moving to a bigger house, or even trying to change your habits can cause stress. This is because there is a major change involved, extra effort is needed, or new responsibilities have come up, and there's a need for adaptation. These circumstances also force us to step into unchartered territory. Wondering how we will deal with these unknowns can be stressful.

Like I mentioned before, not all stress is bad; some of it is beneficial, and it can help save your life or help you perform better. It is the persistently negative response to a stressor that leads to health problems and also affects your wellbeing. However, if you are aware of your stressors and how you react to them, it can help lessen the adverse effects of stress and any negative feelings that might come up.

This is where stress management comes in. It gives you the tools you would need to deal with stressors and resets your internal alarm system. It enables your mind and body to adapt to long-term stress and become more resilient to its effects. Without these tools, your body would always be on high alert, and over time, you would develop chronic stress, which leads to serious health problems.

Causes of Stress

Stress is mainly caused by two things, stressors and your perceptions; it helps to know your stressor so that you can easily manage your stress. Factors or situations that lead to stress are referred to as stressors. Many of us tend to think of stressors as negative, such as a hectic work schedule or a problematic relationship. However, a stressor can be anything that demands a lot from you. This includes positive experiences.

Not all stressors are external factors; sometimes, stress can be self-generated. For instance, when you worry about what others will think of you, fearing change and the unknown, or having irrational, self-defeating thoughts about life, you are experiencing internal stress.

This can include worrying that you will never be good enough, pretty enough, or smart enough.

Your perception of a stressor can also lead to stress. As mentioned before, a stressor to you might not be a stressor to someone else. Take, for instance, how public speaking terrifies some people, while others crave the spotlight. You might thrive under the pressure, while someone else cracks. These different reactions are because of our different perceptions of the situations and how they affect our willpower.

Dealing with Stress

Learning how to handle stress is one of those skills every person needs. After all, stress is inevitable, and you want to be able to handle whatever comes your way. Before we look at a few ways you can deal with stress, you have to understand the different types of stress. Our bodies react to stress depending on whether it is new or short-term, also called acute stress, or whether it has been around for a while in our lives, known as long-term or chronic stress. Let's take a look at each one.

Acute stress

This is temporary stress that comes and goes away quickly, and it's the most common type of stress everyone experiences. It's caused by thinking about the pressure of things or events that have recently happened or that will happen soon. It is an immediate, intense response, and sometimes it can be thrilling due to the release of adrenaline. A good example of this kind of stress is what you feel when you hit the brakes to avoid hitting something or when you have a fast-approaching deadline. Acute stress reduces or completely ends once the stressor is resolved.

A single instance of acute stress is not harmful to your health; it can actually be beneficial and doesn't cause the same amount of damage as long-term stress. However, it can cause tension, headaches, stomach problems, high blood pressure, and other mildly severe health issues.

Repeated instances of acute stress or severe acute stress can cause mental health problems, such as acute stress disorder (ASD) that can eventually lead to chronic stress.

You can develop an acute stress disorder after being exposed to one or many traumatic events. An example of prolonged acute stress disorder is post-traumatic stress disorder (PTSD). Symptoms of ASD can develop after witnessing traumatic or disturbing experiences, such as death or serious injury, firsthand. These symptoms can start or get worse after the traumatic event and can last anywhere between three days and a month. Another form of acute stress is known as episodic acute stress that affects people whose stress triggers are frequent. For instance, if you have too many commitments and poor organizational skills, you can find yourself suffering from episodic acute stress.

Chronic Stress

The other kind of stress is chronic or long-term stress. It's regarded as the most harmful kind of stress because it eats away at you physically, mentally, and emotionally. By the time you realize you have chronic stress, it is too late. Chronic stress can cause burnout if it is not effectively managed because the stress response is triggered all the time, and your body has no time to recover and repair itself before dealing with another wave of stress. This means that your stress response is triggered indefinitely, leaving you in an alarm state all the time.

This type of stress occurs daily, for instance, because you may be stressing over finances, an unhappy marriage, a dysfunctional family, or trouble at work. All these stressors can cause you distress daily because you don't see an end or escape from them. You eventually stop searching for solutions for these problems and resign yourself to your fate.

Chronic stress can continue for a long time and go unnoticed because we become accustomed to the emotions generated and heightened state. This is unlike an episode of acute stress, which is new and often has an immediate solution. This state of chronic stress can become part of your personality because you have never dealt with it, making you more prone to its effects regardless of the situations you might face. Sufferers of chronic stress are more likely to break down and even commit suicide or violent acts as ways of trying to cope with their stress. This is because their willpower is drained and even the slightest pressure can make them crack.

Long-term stress can also cause health issues, such as heart disease, gastrointestinal issues, panic attacks, anxiety, depression, and other medical issues we mentioned before. This is why it's important to manage stress.

Stress Management Techniques

Whether it's acute or chronic stress, your body's stress response is triggered. The only distinction between the two is how long they last. There are numerous techniques you can use to manage stress. Let's take a look at a few:

1. Breathing exercises—these are a great way to calm yourself down and lower your pulse. Once the stress response is activated, your breathing and heart rate will quicken; however, if you stay focused on your breathing and work on getting it back to normal, you will avoid getting into that heightened state. The intake of oxygen will also help you calm your body and mind faster.

Next time you're feeling a bit stressed, you can try this simple breathing technique. Breathe in deeply through the nose, hold it for 5 seconds, then exhale slowly through your mouth. As you inhale, picture yourself breathing in peaceful energy that's getting moved all over your body; when you exhale, you are releasing all the tension and anxiety you might be feeling. Do this until you feel you have calmed down.

2. Progressive muscle relaxation (PMR)—PMR is an effective technique that helps reduce your tension and psychological stress. It involves tensing and relaxing different muscles in your body. By doing this, you are releasing both physical and psychological tension. Research has shown that PMR decreases your stress reactivity and chances of experiencing chronic stress because it helps you recharge your willpower. It is also great for minimizing emotional stress and building resilience.

Simply clench your fist as you inhale, hold for 5 to 10 seconds, then release your hand as you exhale deeply. You can repeat this using different muscle groups such as your face, toes, abdomen, etc. This method works well when combined with a breathing exercise and can be your go-to method for diffusing stressful situations.

3. Mindfulness and meditation—these two techniques are aimed at helping you relax and learn more about yourself. As you meditate and become more mindful, you learn to recognize your thoughts without being judgmental. You also pay attention to your senses and stay focused in the moment. What's great about mindful meditation is you can practice it anywhere. Even 5 minutes at your desk or in the bathroom are enough to calm you down. That said, mastering these practices takes time, but they can greatly impact your life.

While meditating, there are a few tips to keep in mind. Make sure that you are comfortable because small discomforts can distract you from your meditation.

- Don't get too worked up on getting it right, as this can make your meditation more stressful. Instead, let your thoughts enter your mind but focus on redirecting your attention to the present moment rather than dwelling on these thoughts.
- You can play some calming music or use aromatherapy to enhance your meditation. It is optional, though; you do not have to incorporate them; silence works just as well.
- Try and alternate between short and long meditation sessions. You can meditate for about ten to twenty minutes every day and try longer sessions that last thirty minutes or more a few times a week. This will help you improve your meditation and mindfulness techniques and increase your resilience to stress.

4. Exercise—just as with self-control, exercise can help you relieve stress. It is a good way to boost your mood and confidence by providing positive distractions. It can also ease stress symptoms such as anxiety, depression, tension, and fatigue. It's also a great way to work through your feelings and release pent-up energy.

If you are feeling stressed, try doing yoga, tai chi, or boxing.

5. Journal—A journal is a book where you can write down your thoughts and feelings about events in your life. As a stress management technique, it should be done consistently to help you focus on processing emotions and cultivating gratitude. You can write in detail about events happening in your life, your thoughts, feelings, and emotions, and brainstorm solutions to what's bothering you.

You can journal every day or periodically; however, whatever journaling method you choose depends on your personality, the time you have, and doing what feels right to you.

6. Create a support system—whenever you are having a tough time, nothing beats knowing you have someone to talk to. These support systems offer varying types of social support, such as emotional support where you feel that you are listened to and comforted. Moral support is shown through expressions of encouragement and confidence. For instance, your support group can point out the qualities and strengths you forgot you had and let you know they still believe in you.

This boosts your self-confidence because you end up believing in yourself more. Another type of social support you can get is informational support, where you get advice and share information that can help you find out what steps to take when dealing with a particular type of stress. You can also get tangible support, which involves someone else taking over your responsibilities so you can handle your problem. It can also be shown by taking a supportive stand with someone and actively helping them deal with their issues. An example of tangible support would be someone bringing you lunch or dinner when you are ill.

7. Eat well—a healthy diet does more than just fuel your body; it boosts your immunity, gives you energy, replenishes your glucose levels, and can even boost your moods. Whenever you are stressed, you end up having very poor eating habits. For instance, you might skip meals, which causes you to crave unhealthy foods or use food as a coping mechanism. This only leads to more problems; however, by following a healthy diet, you can help your body fight the effects of stress. On that note, you want to cut back on caffeine and alcohol, as they can mess with your sleep patterns. It is crucial that you sleep well.

Other things you can do include listening to music because it calms the soul or playing with your pet. This will help release feel-good hormones and it's also a great mood booster. Managing stress involves using all these strategies to ease the effects stress has on the body. Fortunately, it doesn't have to take stress damaging your health, relationships, or quality of life for you to start practicing stress management techniques.

SIX

How to Stop Procrastinating

PROCRASTINATION IS something everyone has done at some point. You know that feeling you get whenever you don't want to do something even though you know you have to do it, so you put it off until the last possible minute? That's procrastination, and it is an annoyance that hinders you from following through on what you set out to achieve.

Procrastination is a self-regulation problem where we fool ourselves into believing that putting off or avoiding a task will make us feel good. Other times, we overestimate how much time we have to complete the task, how motivated we will be in the future, and how long certain tasks might take. Finally, we assume we will get into the right mindset to complete the task. When we assume tasks won't take as long as they really do, we give ourselves a false sense of hope and security. This false sense of security and waiting to feel inspired to work are the biggest contributors to procrastination.

Simply waiting until you are in the right frame of mind to do something, especially if it's something you are dreading, doesn't work. You will find that the right time never seems to come, meaning there's a high chance the tasks will remain incomplete. Another major contributor to this procrastination habit is self-doubt. If you are unsure or don't know how to handle a particular task, you can start doubting your skills and end up putting it off as you tackle other easier tasks first.

According to research, about 20 percent of all American adults are chronic procrastinators. They don't just occasionally postpone things; procrastination is a major part of their lifestyle. Here's how: they pay their bills late, get to work late, start working on major projects just as the deadline approaches, and even wait until Christmas Eve to do their Christmas shopping. Unfortunately, this procrastination behavior can have adverse effects on your mental health.

A 2007 study of college students showed that, at the start of the semester, chronic procrastinators had lower stress levels and related illnesses since there were no looming deadlines. However, toward the end of the semester, their stress levels were very high and they had other stress-related issues such as high blood pressure or anxiety. As you can see, procrastination can have severe effects on your health and social life as well.

You may find that there are things you want to accomplish, but your procrastination habits are holding you back. You have no clue where to start or what needs to be done; you lack the initiative to get started because you are waiting for the right moment. All this can create a mental hurdle that's too big to get over. If, for example, you want to start a business, but you don't have the capital or the technical know-how, this can force you to put your plans on the back burner as you wait to get enough money or enough knowledge on where and how to start.

To get your new business off the ground, start off by educating yourself if you are unfamiliar with what you want to venture into. Let's say that real estate was what you chose because you love it, but you have no idea how to get into it. A logical step would be to get educated about real estate. To become a real estate agent, one must first take the real estate licensing educational course and pass the real estate licensing exam, which shows that you are competent enough to be selling houses. Once you are educated, you need to learn how to sell real estate; this includes tips and tricks. This is where networking comes in handy. Learn from your peers and mentors, too, and get to know how they got there. Once you learn how to sell property, you will eventually learn how to close deals faster and thus be a step closer to achieving your ultimate goal of being rich.

The first step is having a system to help you stay on track with what you are working on at the time. Research shows that people tend to focus better and are more energetic for longer periods when they work for about 90 minutes and then take a 30-minute break. The real trick, however, was to know what to do during this break. Whatever you choose to do during this break is important because you have to maintain your productivity levels, as well as keep the urge to procrastinate away.

For instance, do a few, short pleasurable tasks such as walking your dog, meditating, or doing some yoga stretches. Avoid checking your social media accounts. They can easily drain your energy and trap you in a spiral of procrastination. You need to keep your mind alert and ready for when you go back to your project.

The second step is practicing mindfulness because no matter how hard or diligent a worker you might be, everyone hits a slump, and their minds wander once in a while. What's important is the ability to recognize that your mind is wandering and bring back your focus to the task at hand. For instance, if during an intense workout you found yourself thinking how sore your whole body is and you would rather be resting, understand it's totally normal to feel this way. However, if you want to achieve your weight loss goals, you have to rein in these thoughts.

Don't let them bring your spirits down; instead, you can use them as motivation. Tell yourself it's only going to hurt for a while, and hold onto the image of how good you will look in the end. By using mindful meditation through this lapse in motivation, you can acknowledge that your mind has wandered from the task at hand and also take note of the thoughts and feelings that have erupted from working out. Take a deep breath, let go of these thoughts, then use your mindfulness to bring back your attention to where you need it to be.

Lastly, aside from your to-do-list, create another list of all the tasks you have completed. Think of it as your victory list. It will serve as a log of everything you have accomplished and also as a reinforcement system for all your positive efforts. Remember, everything doesn't have to be perfect. Believe in yourself and what you have done and it will be enough. Don't be afraid of failure because, without it, we can never learn.

Staying Motivated in Life and Work

Achieving your goals is never easy, and knowing how to stay motivated can make all the difference. Today's world is riddled with distractions that can easily capture your attention. From exposure to social media to texts and emails that keep coming in, you may be getting increasingly unfocused and unproductive. Lacking motivation can lead to procrastination, which can cause you to put your plans on hold permanently. Some days, you get up and you're ready to go, and other times you can barely get out of bed because you lack that intrinsic drive.

Keeping yourself motivated can be hard, even under the best circumstances. So how do you stay pumped when you just quit your job to follow your passion, but you have no inkling where to begin or when things at home are getting out of hand because you are so busy, you forgot to do the chores? You have probably heard of those directives to put a picture of yourself at your fittest on your dresser or plaster affirmations such as "You are the best," or "You can do it," all over the house, but motivation isn't like magic. You can't buy it in a bottle or swallow a pill to get motivated; it is an energy that you tap into and harness by design.

Motivation is derived from the word motive, which refers to the wants, desires, or drives of a person. It is the process of stimulating a person to act and accomplish their goals. Motivators can be things like money, success, and emotions like pride. Motivation is influenced by the fulfillment of needs that are either required for the sustenance of life or essential for wellbeing or growth. Psychological needs of belonging, mastery over one's life, and autonomy guide our behavior along the same lines as our need for achievement, power, closure, finding meaning, gaining confidence, and self-esteem. All these make up the internal motives for most of the activities we engage in. Our social context, goals, values, desires, and environment play a big role as external motivators.

An athlete training hard to run a mile in under six minutes or a sick person working hard to lose weight and strengthen his body are simple examples of reasons why some people would work out. The athlete is motivated by achievement, while the sick person is motivated by the need to be healthy. So, to understand how to stay motivated, you must know what motivates you. What drives you to want to achieve that goal you have set out? Once these reasons are clear in your mind, you can use these tips to stay motivated.

Break down your goals further and visualize as much detail as you can. See what you want to achieve clearly in your mind; think of how it will feel. Visualize every single detail of the goal you have set forth. By doing so, you will be conditioning your body to live in the future, preparing yourself for when you will achieve your goal. Take, for instance, deciding you want to run a marathon. As you practice, visualize the performance, how you will run, how your body will feel. Imagine how the breeze will feel on your face, your chest pounding, the sweat dripping, and the cheers from the crowds as you cross the finish line. Keep that picture in your mind as vividly as possible and use it to re-energize you in those moments you feel tired or want to give up.

Make a list of the reasons why this goal is important to you. You have to stay grounded in your goal. Take out a piece of paper and a pen and write down your goal and all the reasons you can come up with why this goal is so important to you. Don't type them out, but rather write them down because writing engages the brain more and you can really get into what you are doing. This deeper mental connection can help you jog up memories of things you had forgotten as you write your reasons down.

If you have a goal, break it down into smaller ones, and set targets and rewards. A big part of why many people lose motivation once they set out to achieve a goal is because they often underestimate the scope of everything they have to do. Even a simple goal, such as being happy, involves a lot of moving parts, which, if not dealt with correctly, can cause you to fail. When you feel like you have a lot on your plate, you can easily get stressed and overwhelmed and fail or quit what you are doing.

If you have chosen to take on a project no matter the size, break it down into smaller, more realistic goals and tackle one at a time. If you say you want to change your life, this in itself is a grand undertaking; where do you start? Break down your life-changing goal into smaller goals such as you will get your finances in order, love life, and care for your physical and mental health. And you can further break down these sub-goals to create a detailed plan of how you will ultimately change your life.

Establish a reward system for yourself. It is always delightful to be compensated for all of your hard work and effort and you can benefit greatly from having a reward system in place. After you achieve a small goal, reward yourself. This releases feel-good hormones, which will motivate you to keep going. The reward doesn't have to be extravagant; even small treats can prove to be great rewards. Play around with various types of rewards and reward systems to see what works best for you.

Schedule in breaks. Trying to achieve goals can easily overwhelm even the most determined people; when you feel like you are burning out, it is time to take a well-deserved break. Breaks give you time to recuperate your energy and also to refocus. If your goal, for instance, is fitness-related, you cannot do much once you are exhausted, so take an extended rest of three to five days instead of the usual two-day break you would normally have between workout sessions. If you are learning something new, don't try to learn it all in one sitting. Pace yourself and allocate time to review what you have learned.

Get a strategy and be ready to change course if needed. Failure can be the biggest demotivator, but you have to be prepared for it. Our greatest weakness lies in giving up instead of getting up and trying again. Always have a contingency plan in place in case things don't go your way. As you plan, your plans must accommodate failures, setbacks, and temporary defeats. These temporary roadblocks serve as lessons and chances for you to stop and reevaluate and see what you might be doing wrong. Take it easy on yourself if you fail. It is part of the process. Take it as a lesson, but don't dwell on it; accept it and continue working toward your goals. Take on what you need to do next with renewed zeal to help you overcome the slump caused by your recent failure.

Be aware of when you require help and get it. There is value in announcing your intentions to others. It conveys a strong message to the world and, more importantly, to your subconscious mind, which can sometimes hamper our efforts. We often overestimate our abilities and can fall short, so learn to seek help. You might be surprised by what you might gain. However, be very selective of who you tell about your goals or whom you ask for help because not everyone will give you good advice.

Finding the motivation to do this thing that is important to us sometimes isn't as simple as it would seem. We must think about whether it is competing with other motives, whether internal or external, and take stock of our values to ensure they don't clash. For external motivators, we may have to intervene in how they influence our motivation to make sure they match our internal levels. To be successful in motivating ourselves or even others, our internal motives must match our external motives.

Find the Right Mentors

After identifying your goal, you must push yourself to find, talk, and engage with those that have already achieved that goal. You need to surround yourself with mentors and peers and learn from them. You may know some of them, and others may be strangers to you; you might even dislike some of them, but if they have something that you have identified as beneficial to you, you must learn from them to get to where they are. Working in conjunction with a mentor can increase your chances of succeeding fivefold. However, it doesn't mean that you should take every mentoring opportunity that comes your way. Take time to analyze the opportunity, your ability to commit, and your potential mentor. Selecting the right mentor is critical to helping you grow and achieve your goals.

A mentor is an experienced, trusted advisor. However, they are more than that. They are three things: consultants, counselors, and cheerleaders. As consultants, they offer advice, insight, and wisdom gained through real-world experiences. They are often experienced in areas that you are seeking help for and can be an invaluable resource to you. As counselors, they listen and offer guidance, often leading you halfway to the answer, so that they can figure the rest out for yourself. Instead of pointing out mistakes, they offer valuable lessons using those mistakes along the way. As cheerleaders, they offer support, enthusiasm, and constructive feedback. Mentors should celebrate your successes no matter how big or small because the journey is full of ups and downs, and encouragement is vital.

Mentorship can take on various forms, from one-on-one relationships to a mentoring group in an organization, but the best mentoring relationships are where both parties learn from each other.

When picking out your mentor, you need to determine exactly what you need. Ask yourself, at the stage you are at, what skills do you need to learn now versus 6-months or a year from now? The path to achieving your goals is never linear and the mentor you get right now might not have the skills to help you along two years from now. That is why it is important to examine your current developmental needs before looking at future ones.

- Weigh their strengths and weaknesses and how they relate to your needs and style. You don't have to change your whole working style to accommodate someone else's teaching. It would be too exhausting. When picking out a mentor, check whether their style clashes with yours. You want to find someone who thinks like you, has skills you want to emulate, and has similar qualities to you because it will be easier to learn from them. Take time to find out if your world views, values, and outlooks are aligned.

Focus on things such as learning, determination, thoughtfulness, trust, and other similar values. Take time to study your potential mentor so you can set your expectations accordingly.

- Your mentor must be a good listener. Mentors and mentees travel different paths. Even if they have gone through similar challenges, they should not spoon-feed you the answers. Rather, they should listen to you and help you overcome your challenges by guiding you to find your own way. You should develop your own mind and senses with your mentor being but a guide.

A mentor should also listen to your ideas, not just your problems. They should advise you when you can go for it or give you a reality check without dashing your hopes.

- Your mentor should challenge you. First, you have to disregard the notion that mentors have to be people older than you. This is outdated thinking because a mentor can be anyone who is experienced and trusted in that particular area. That being said, you won't learn much from your mentor if they don't get you to consider new perspectives. Since you should ideally share the same philosophies, think of how you share ideas.

You want someone who has had similar experiences but also someone who took different approaches to overcome them—someone who teaches by challenging your beliefs and stances and not someone who shoots down ideas prematurely.

- Master the art of asking someone to be your mentor. Once you have identified an individual who fits all your criteria, find a way to ask them to be your mentor. Being a mentor is a big ask, and not everyone will be in a position to take on mentees.

But if they agree to take you on, you have to take some initiative to help this relationship grow. Initiate contact, ask them for feedback, persevere, and commit to the process.

- When you are around people that have accomplished what you want to achieve, you will eventually begin to see what they see. Once you begin to view the world the same way they do and see their reality, you will ultimately get closer to reaching your goal. Your vision is not cloudy anymore. You understand the work ethic, desire, sacrifice, and determination it takes to get to where you want. By working with a mentor and other peers, it will push you to a level of unimaginable growth. Everything is in your hands and you will finally be able to make your reality come true.

SEVEN

How to Maintain Good Habits Every Day

A HABIT IS something you constantly do and is often unconscious. No matter how small the habit might be, such as biting your nails, it can be incredibly powerful. Your habits are the compound interest of your self-improvement. If you want better results, forget about setting goals but rather focus on creating a good system. Remember the habit formation process? That's the same system all habits and behaviors follow. So if you want to modify your habits to make good ones, the only way to help them stick is by ensuring the habit formation process works in your favor.

In his book, *Atomic Habits*, James Clear breaks down behavioral change into 4 simple rules that you can use to build good habits. Start by making the cue obvious, the trigger attractive, the response easy, and the reward satisfying. By grasping these simple rules, you can make any habit easily stick. The most important thing to remember is while getting good behavior is your end goal; it shouldn't be your main focus. You want to put a lot more effort into the system because it will lead to these results.

Tips to Help you Stick with Good Habits

So, how do you stick to good habits every day? Here are a few practical tips to help you along.

1. Use visual cues—in 1993, when Trent Dyrsmid was 23, he was hired by a bank in Abbotsford. As a rookie, no one expected much from him. That's why his success story is so fascinating. Each morning he placed 2 jars on his desk: one filled with 120 paper clips and the other empty. After settling in, he would start making sales calls, and after he was done with one call, he moved a clip into the empty jar.

He made these calls until he moved all the clips to the empty jar. Within a year and a half of working at the bank, he brought in about $5 million to the firm. By the age of 25, he was making $75,000 a year, which is about $125,000 in today's money. Soon after, he was hired by another company and moved on to making even more money. So how did he become so successful? Simple, he created a winning system. Each morning after getting to work, he would start making calls and never stopped until he was done.

In the beginning, we all commit to our various goals; however, we never really think about the systems we have in place to achieve these goals. How are we going to stay on track? How are we going to get started? For instance, we know we should eat healthier, but why don't we?

The difference between Trent and the rest of us is that he created a system to help him achieve his goals. The paperclips served as a visual cue urging him to make those calls. Visual cues help remind you to start a behavior. They serve as an extrinsic reminder of what we need to do. Many times we overestimate our ability to remember to stick to a new habit. After all, your subconscious has the biggest say in it, so you will fail if you don't make a conscious effort.

Visual cues also serve as displays of your progress. Take Trent's paper clips, for instance. They showed him how many calls he had made and how many he needed to make. This can be quite useful, especially in building consistency. As you start your journey to change and stick to good habits, take some time to find your paper clips. They can be anything you want, such as balls, marbles, pins, cards, etc.—just remember to keep it simple, though.

Lastly, visual cues can have an additive effect on motivation. As you see your progress, you get more motivated to keep up the habit. The more paper clips in your completed jar, the more value they have. This effect is referred to as the "endowed progress effect." It states that you are more likely to place more value on things once you have them. This means the more clips you move to the completed jar, the more valuable completing the task will be.

2. Be consistent—the trick to getting good habits on autopilot is creating a system that makes it easy to adopt new habits. The key to developing this system is consistency. Before a new behavior can become automatic, you need to repeat it consistently for it to stick.

For instance, if you want to be more grateful, you have to find ways to show gratitude every day, even when you feel there's nothing to be grateful about. If you make it through this conditioning phase, your new behavior will be much easier to manage and sustain. Once you get used to doing things daily, it's a lot easier to turn them into habits.

3. Start simple—if you are looking to foster more self-love in your life, you can't start off trying to completely change everything about yourself; it won't work. You need to start simple and small; after all, it took years for these self-hating habits to form. What makes you think you can change them overnight? Real change takes time because you have a long way to go.

If you aimed too big, you might get over-motivated and take on too much, go too fast, and run out of steam midway. However, if you pace yourself, you have a better chance of developing a working system because building on what you have bit by bit will help you make a bigger change. Take, for instance, exercising. Working out intensely for 2 hours on the first day might seem easy, but it will leave you really sore the next day, which might demotivate you from working out more. However, if you started with 30-minute sessions and worked your way up to an hour, you are more likely to stick to training because your body isn't overworked.

4. Remind yourself of your goals—as you work on changing, you can easily lose sight of why you started doing all this along the way. The daily rigors of effecting the change could easily distract you from your main goal.

That's why it's important to constantly remind yourself of the end goal and the commitment you made. Try putting up stickers to remind you of your goals on your fridge or dresser.

5. Get an accountability partner—while on your journey of change, it's easy to deviate from the track since you have no one holding you accountable. You think it's okay if you miss a few days at the gym to rest because you will get back on track afterwards.

However, this can lead you down a path of procrastination which eventually demotivates you from doing what you set out to. That's why getting an accountability buddy is so crucial. They can help you stay on track even when your motivation wanes.

6. Accept failure—if there's one thing that holds true in life, it is that failure is part of life. There's no way around it. You have to fail to succeed, so don't expect all your attempts at change to succeed immediately. You might fail more times than you like, but that's the beauty of it. Through this failure, you will learn what you need to change to make it work. For instance, you might start going to the gym a bunch of times before you get consistent. So don't strive for perfection. You are human and real change takes time, so accept your imperfections, and you will have an easier time. This is why adopting a growth mindset is key.

Habits That Might Keep You from Sticking to Good Habits

- Comparisons—in life, it's an inevitability that you will compare yourself with others at some point. You will often find yourself lacking, which can trigger feelings of anger, low self-esteem, and inadequacy. That's why when you see other people living happy lives, you feel envious. That said, you can have what's known as a healthy social comparison. This isn't about seeing yourself as a failure but using your ability to find out what it is you admire in others and imitating those admirable qualities or even improving on them.

The best comparison you can make, however, is with yourself. Take a look at your past and see where you were. Are you at a better place now than you were in the past? What can you do to improve yourself further?

- Maximization—have you ever found yourself not going for something because you are waiting for a better deal? Have you ever bought something and think, I bet I could have gotten a better deal on this? Maximizers search for better deals even when they have already gotten what they need. It is crucial to distinguish between what we want and what we need. Oftentimes, we are better off with just getting what we need rather than getting what we want.

Maximizers lose out on the opportunities to be present in their lives and enjoy the good moments they have. They also have very little gratitude because you can't be thankful if you aren't satisfied, right?

- Perfectionism—first off, we can never be perfect, so the pursuit of perfection pits you against your own nature. How could you be happy or content? Perfectionism is often mistaken for meticulousness, which involves having attainable and tangible expectations. Perfectionism, on the other hand, involves having unrealistic levels of expectations and intangible goals. Perfectionists often have the all-or-nothing mindset, often only seeing things in black and white rather than in reality's colorful splendor.

When things don't go their way or are not to their standards, they view themselves as failures, which makes them failures. Trying to attain perfection only creates problems. Is it even worth it? That said, always strive to do your best. Attaining perfection is nearly impossible, but it doesn't mean you should abandon all pursuits. Instead, think of them as a journey rather than the final destination, and every action you do that yields results as a learning opportunity.

- Materialism—you've heard it countless times; attaching your self-worth or happiness to material things is a dangerous game to play.

What if you got fired and you can't sustain that lifestyle? What then?

- Overgeneralization—this refers to holding every experience you had to be true and applicable to every other experience every time. For example, your last relationship ended badly, so you apply that experience to other blossoming relationships and conclude you will never have a good one. The thing with overgeneralization is it views failure as the end of the world and closes you off to trying things again. Remember, this journey to happiness is hard, and failing is part of it.

However, if you hold onto these failures and say that you will fail every time you try, you most definitely will because you won't even try, and that's the sure-fire way to ensure your failure 100 percent. Would the odds be better if, instead of 100 percent guaranteeing failure by not trying to at least try with a chance of 10 percent success or even 1 percent? That's still better than 0 percent when you don't even try.

- Downplaying your wins—finding ways to downplay your positive moments like they don't count, saying it was luck or you failed less than others.

You need to acknowledge your successes.

- Skewing your reality— this involves assuming what you are feeling is always a representation of reality. "I made a mistake during my presentation. Everyone must think I am a fool."

But in reality, do they? Most likely they didn't even notice.

- Jumping to negative conclusions—making leaps to negative conclusions without any evidence to support your claim. "I know something is going to go wrong."

You act like you are suddenly psychic and know what will happen, or like you can read minds, "I know they will hate me." How can you know for sure?

- Letting past mistakes define you—defining yourself based on your past mistakes or perceived lack of skills. An example is saying you are not smart enough because you failed at something before or thinking that you could never achieve the same success as others and refusing to try things out because you think you will fail.

Success is a result of committing to the basics over and over again. That's why creating a working system is so important. It will help you stick to your fundamentals through the highs and the lows. Sticking to good habits goes way beyond willpower; it requires you to adopt a system that sets you up for success. Remember, creating good habits isn't the overall goal, since habits are a means to an end. What's important is understanding the role they play in the pursuit of success.

EIGHT

Overcoming Challenges—Keep Pushing Forward Even If You Fail

SOMETIMES THINGS GO PRETTY WELL, or even better than that, and other times they go horribly wrong. Making a mistake or failing isn't fun. It hurts and can be so devastating that you consider quitting whatever it is you were doing. However, these setbacks or challenges are part of everyday life. They are an inescapable and unavoidable part of being human. So, if they are not going anywhere, how do we deal with them? How do you pick yourself up when you are feeling completely devastated?

Contrary to popular belief, failure is not the opposite of success. For far too long, we've been fed this narrative that failure cannot coexist with success and that it is the enemy, something that should be avoided at all costs. And so, we have strived to avoid failure in everything we do. But everyone fails. It's inevitable; in fact, we probably fail at something every day. Does it mean that we are failures?

A lot of successful people faced challenges and failed countless times before they became a success. There's no success story that wasn't founded in failure. How many times did Babe Ruth strike out before he made record home runs? How many KFC recipes failed before they got the right one? How many shots did Jordan miss before he became the GOAT (the greatest of all time)? He lost over three hundred games in his career and missed 9,000 shots; 26 times, his teammates trusted him to take the game-winning shot but he missed, costing them the game. Despite all this, he is regarded as the greatest basketball player of all time.

Walt Disney, the guy behind so many lovable characters such as Mickey and Minnie, was told he had no creativity. His first company, Laugh-O-Gram, failed after a partner pulled out. Desperate and out of money, he faced a lot of ridicule, failure, and criticism before his first few films became famous, and the Disney company that you know today was born.

When you form a company, job security isn't something you worry about. In his twenties, Steve Jobs found success when Apple became a huge hit. However, in his thirties, the company's board of directors fired him. Unfazed by the failure, he founded a new company, NeXT, that was eventually acquired by Apple. Once back at his old company, he proved his capacity for success by reinventing Apple.

Michael Jordan, Babe Ruth, Colonel Sanders, Steve Jobs, and a lot of other successful people have failed massively, sometimes so badly that it looked like the end of their careers. Do you think they let these failures or setbacks get them down?

Whenever we fail, our expectations are dashed. In that moment, failure seems like the end, but it's not. How you perceive it is what matters. Admitting that failure is part of the learning process can help reduce the fear and anxiety that it causes. It can also reduce the negative self-reflection that we are bad because we failed. Failing means we get to learn something new. It means that we tried to do something new, embraced change, and helped prepare for success.

For most of us, success is our only motivator; the better we are at something, the more motivated we are to keep doing it. However, life isn't so easy. If you hinge your motivation on success, you will have a hard time dealing with setbacks and challenges. The biggest motivator of really successful people is failure. Failure gives them an opportunity to learn and do better next time. They use failure as a ladder to success.

If you were to talk to these people, you would discover they have also faced numerous setbacks, failures, and challenges. For many of us, one failure is enough to put us off. You often hear people saying," It wasn't meant to be," or "At least we tried. That's good enough." They move on to the next thing, hoping it will go well because if it doesn't, they can't move on; they get stuck in a slump.

Understand that failure is part of life and success is not a straight line. You will face setbacks, roadblocks, devastating defeats, and other challenges as you work towards your goals. The key, however, is not getting lost in the haze but staying focused on the end goal. So how do you overcome challenges?

First, understand the different obstacles you will face

Failure, setbacks, challenges, roadblocks, and obstacles all represent things that will get in your way. While they are grouped together, each represents a different level of challenge. Setbacks, for instance, are relatively minor hiccups that occur along the way. Think of them like speed bumps on a road that you don't need to stop your vehicle for, just drive slowly. They will slow you down. These are problems that make it harder for you to accomplish what you set out to do.

After setbacks come roadblocks; just as the name implies, these challenges do more than slow you down; they stop you in your tracks. You can think of them as quicksand. They actually pose a greater threat to your progress because you can get stuck, which impedes your progress. Unlike setbacks, roadblocks leave lasting effects. For instance, if you were working on a project due on Friday and your computer crashed on Tuesday night, you are likely to miss your deadline.

Even if you turn in your work on Monday, your boss or the client will still be unhappy about the delay. Even though you might not lose your job, you might not be the go-to guy anymore. Your boss might assign you less important work until you can be trusted again. However, you can still bounce back from this.

After roadblocks come defeats or failures. This is when you give something your all and it blows in your face. Unlike the other two kinds of challenges, defeats leave you wondering what you will do next. Think of them as total knockouts. You are left reeling on the ground, often still in shock.

Why Failure Has a Bad Reputation

While I'm all for trying and failing, understand that there are real consequences to failing. Not succeeding can be disappointing and painful. To make it worse, we as a society have glorified winning and demonized failing, such that we only celebrate our successes and not the struggles we go through to achieve them. Winning isn't everything; it only becomes the only thing. With this all-or-nothing mindset, we take on life with a closed view. We either win or lose, and losers are never remembered. But life is not like that. It's full of ups and downs and you can't be up every time.

Other than the disappointment and pain we feel when we fail, there are other hidden consequences that run deeper and are more damaging and crippling. These consequences matter because they impact our future efforts and how we feel about ourselves. Whenever we face failure, two things happen:

- We shut down because the shame of falling weighs on us like an anvil and feels like a hammer to the head. We close ourselves off to challenges and new ideas. We basically stop learning.
- We view failure as something that must be avoided at all costs. But this is impossible, given that failure is a part of the learning process. This misconstrued view of failure causes us to stop trying because if we don't try, we can't fail.

When this happens, we internalize the fear of failure, which spawns a vicious cycle of procrastination and avoidance. Let's think of an example. Dan was terrified that he wouldn't get a job after college. His fear of failing to get the right job made him delay applying for jobs and he missed out on some great opportunities. His peers, on the other hand, applied for and got these jobs. Now he felt ashamed that he failed to start working on time just like his peers did. This led to further procrastination. There was a career center at the college where Dan went; however, he never used it. His fear kept him trapped and unable to use all the resources available to him.

Do you see how important it is not to fear failure?

That's what fearing failure does. It traps you in this cocoon where you are trapped with all these negative emotions, such as shame and disappointment. You close your mind off to everything available to you. Had Dan gone to the career center, he would have gotten the help he needed and probably landed a job. When we choose to try something new, our fear of getting it wrong can be crippling. It hinders our ability to learn, be present, and give it our best shot. Instead, we are preoccupied with what-ifs.

What if we fail? What then? These what-ifs convince us to wait for the perfect conditions, which unfortunately don't happen. We create a self-fulfilling prophecy where our fear of failure leads us to put off practicing, participating, or getting help, thus increasing our chances of failing. It's like we want to fail. We then generalize ourselves as failures and spiral into hopelessness and even despair.

Perks of Failure

The Oxford dictionary defines failure as "not being successful." Then, it's divided into "countable" and "uncountable" definitions. The uncountable definition describes it as "the lack of success in doing or achieving something." Alternatively, the countable version describes it as a "person or thing that is not successful." Simple enough, right? However, somewhere along the line, we misconstrued this simple definition and derived our own translation.

We define our own failure as being a let-down, unworthy, and useless person. How did we get all that from the dictionary definition? This definition alone shows that failure isn't as bad as we think. In fact, it is actually good for us. Interesting, isn't it? Think of failure as a good thing. As we move on, I want you to think of failure as "a different than anticipated result that is not necessarily bad."

Here are a few benefits of failure:

It provides a reality check

Nothing transports us back to reality faster than failure. When you fail, you are devastated. But failing allows you to look back at the whole situation in a new light. Let's see another example. Ever since Jonah was 12, he dreamt of going to college. If he made it, he'd be the first member of his family to ever go to college. He knew that if he didn't get good grades, he'd lose his chance. On top of that, his career advisor often told him that he wasn't academic enough to get into college. He, however, did not let this bring him down. He decided to take AP classes to improve his grades; however, Jonah failed. He never made it to college.

Why? Why did Jonah fail despite wanting this more than anything else? There's a simple answer and that is that he wasn't in the right frame of mind. The added pressure from the extra classes, being told that he was not academic enough, and his whole family's hopes and dreams hinging on this made him think that failure was not an option. All this had a bad effect on his studies and eventually resulted in him failing. Sometimes failing at something, even if you truly desire it, serves as an indicator that something isn't right somewhere else. Failure helps reveal what's really going on in your situation.

It's a learning experience

Failure is a great, somewhat harsh teacher. In your life, career, finances, and life goals, learning what not to do is just as crucial as learning what to do. You can't have one without the other. Failure leaves you room to right yourself and allows you to learn from your mistakes. This helps you recommit to your goals because now you know what to do from having learned what not to do through failure.

· · ·

It builds character

When you fail, you gain insight into yourself and the task at hand. Anyone can be the hero in good times but how do you measure up when the going gets tough? Does the pressure get to you and you crumble or do you stand your ground and keep fighting? While failure can shake us to our core, going through it tests your character, courage, determination, and mindset. Without it, you can't truly appreciate your best. It serves as a benchmark to show you what you are made of, which is, hopefully, steel.

It fosters creativity and innovation

Failure opens you up to more probabilities and approaches. You are not afraid to think outside the box because failure pushes you to re-evaluate your goals and efforts. When we fail, we get the chance to try again and implement what we learned from our failed attempts. We don't live in a one-shot-only world and the problems we face often require creative solutions. There's no clear-cut path to success; we have to adapt it to our unique situations. Fail, fail, and fail again. That way, you figure out what works and what doesn't and can find creative solutions to getting things done and getting there.

It makes you more resilient

Failure can deal some pretty painful blows. However, it's impossible to live without failure. Doing so will make you cautious of everything. What kind of life is that? And won't you, in essence, fail at living? You didn't learn how to ride a bicycle without falling off a couple of times. You'll probably get a lot of scratches and scrapes, but after failing over and over again, you'll get the hang of it. Failing helps develop resilience. Learning from your failures helps you recover quicker. After falling off the bike, you know what to do to stay on. It makes you stronger, so you can easily face any new challenges. Keep moving forward and keep fighting despite the setbacks you face.

Fearing failure is worse than failure itself

Fear, fear, fear. It seems like everything that keeps us from achieving our goals is fear-related; fear of the future, fear of change, fear of failure, and so on. There's no real alternative to failure; you can choose to try something new and have a 50 percent chance of failing or not try it at all and be sure to fail 100 percent. If you genuinely want to be happier, you have to change some things, and that leaves you open to failure. Even though you don't know how it will turn out, you need to try out new things and take risks. When you fail, you will get a chance to learn from your failure. This means that you can take intelligent risks next time and increase your chances of success. The fear of failing prevents you from trying, which is the biggest failure of all.

Coping with Failure and Challenges

Learning how to cope with failure takes some of the fear out of failing. It makes it easier to embrace it and even reduces the pain you feel so you can bounce back better than before. Failure allows you to appreciate where you are in your journey, even if it's not where you wanted to be. Every failure has its purpose. Learn from it. Here are various ways you can cope with failure and everything it brings into your life.

1. Don't take the failure personally

If nothing else sticks, remember this one. Don't take failure personally. Everyone fails; it's part of the success process, and there's no way around it. You must learn to separate failure from your personal identity. Failure is not a trait you have; it's a part of life. Just because the idea you had failed, it doesn't mean you are a failure. Failing comes with a lot of emotions, and if you take them all to heart, bouncing back from it becomes a momentous task. Failure is not about your value as a person. It doesn't change your overall worth to your family, friends, or community. It's simply showing what works and what doesn't so you can change accordingly.

2. Ask yourself why you failed

To move forward from failure, we must know what went wrong in the first place. If not, how are we going to figure out what we need to change? Take, for example, a job presentation; when it doesn't go according to plan, take some time and reflect on it. Did you cover everything you needed to? Did you have the right team backing you up? Did you do enough research? Whatever the reason for the failure is, find out what it is so that you can make the necessary changes, or else you are doomed to repeat your failure.

3. Handle your emotions

A lot of emotions accompany failure: anxiety, shame, embarrassment, anger, sadness, etc. These are uncomfortable feelings, and we will do anything to escape from them. Remember, our minds are wired to avoid pain, and if failure causes pain, then our brains will work extra hard to keep us from feeling that discomfort. A study published in the *Journal of Behavioral Decision Making* showed that we shouldn't try to brush off or avoid dealing with the feelings elicited by failure.

Dealing with your emotions will help you recognize any unhealthy attempts to reduce pain. Not dealing with the emotions you have causes you to find other ways to distract yourself from the pain and fill the void with food, drugs, love, an unhealthy obsession with money or looks. However, these things won't heal your pain; they only provide temporary relief.

By mindfully reflecting on these, we can learn a lot about ourselves. Embrace that anger, disappointment, and sadness you feel. When things don't go your way, have a good cry, feel the emotions; don't try to fight or ignore them. Afterwards, make yourself a drink and take the edge off. You'll be able to see things more clearly now. Allowing yourself to feel bad about your failure can serve as motivation. It can push you to work harder and find better solutions, so you will be better next time.

4. Be brutally honest and take responsibility

Take a long hard look at yourself. Mostly when we fail, we are quick to try and fix the situation rather than reflect on what happened. Distractions can derail us from self-reflection in the wake of failure; however, this is a significant part of the process. We hate confronting ourselves about our mistakes, yet this is the only way we can learn from them. When we are honest about what happened, we can own up to our mistakes. We are able to find explanations and identify the reasons behind the failure and the part we played in it, rather than coming up with excuses and blaming others.

5. Practice healthy stress coping skills

Call a trusted friend, practice some deep breathing techniques, take a relaxing bubble bath, play some music, or dance. These are a few examples of how you can cope with stress healthily. When handling stress, it's all about finding what works for you. Failing can be stressful and if you struggle with bad habits whenever you are stressed, such as drinking or smoking, they can worsen. Create a list of healthy stress coping skills and techniques you can use and place them somewhere you can easily see them. Use this list to remind you that there are healthier strategies you can turn to whenever you are feeling bad.

6. Make adjustments

After coming to terms with everything, including the fact that you failed and why you failed, ask yourself, what can I adjust to make things better? Did I set very high expectations? Or maybe I didn't give it all I could? Whatever it may be, failure is a learning opportunity. Find out what you need to change and make sure you don't make the same mistake again. Failing isn't bad, but failing the same way over and over again is.

7. Fail forward

You fail forward by studying your mistakes and setbacks. Look at what you can learn and make the necessary arrangements when creating a plan to move forward. If you are open to learning, failure can be a great teacher. Did you make one mistake or a series of them that ultimately led to your failure? What can you do differently next time? Even as you think of all this, don't keep replaying your failures in your head. If you allow yourself to ruminate on everything that went wrong, you'll get stuck in this black hole of despair and hopelessness. Fail forward; see where you went wrong and factor this in when creating a plan to move forward.

8. Be realistic about your goals and failure

Our expectations can set us up. We must always create realistic expectations and SMART goals. We are more likely to sabotage ourselves when we are convinced that one mistake makes us a total failure. It can be easy to think that tossing your goals out would solve the problem. However, that would be a horrific misunderstanding of the intentions of this book. I'm not saying don't set any goals, just be SMART about them.

SMART goals should be **S**pecific, **M**easurable, **A**chievable, **R**ealistic, and **T**ime-bound. I want you to focus on the realistic part. Don't go aiming for the moon, then hate yourself for falling short. If you do aim for the moon and fail, it's okay. You actually succeeded. Take failure as part of the process, and accept all the irrational beliefs you have about it. These often feed your fear of failure. To remind yourself to have more realistic thoughts about failure, remember:

- Failure shows you are challenging yourself.
- Don't take it personally.
- You can handle failing; after all, it's a great opportunity to learn.
- Repeat these declarations over and over again to help you remain realistic about failure and bounce back.

We cannot stop obstacles from materializing in our lives, but we can choose how to handle them. In your pursuit of self-love and change, you are bound to face many failures along the way. Don't be afraid of failing. Changing your habits is not easy, nor is sticking to good habits; a lot of the parts of this journey are hard and you will fail. However, this shouldn't stop you from pushing on. You might discover new opportunities and even learn to see yourself in a more positive light and not as the loser you always thought you were.

Doing the Most with Least Effort

In a world where things get harder by the day, it seems we are all looking for a more effortless way to get things done. On a fundamental level, we are all lazy, and we can't help it. That's why we will always choose the easiest way to do something or try to put it off for as long as possible. Ever found yourself saying," I'll definitely get that assignment done later on." or "I'm too tired. There's got to be an easier way to get this done?" These sentiments are nothing new and are something you share with billions of people on earth.

Take a look at everything we have covered so far, such as practicing self-love, changing your habits, or even building your willpower. They all require a notable amount of effort to pull off. Doing a task depletes your energy, and the amount of energy you expend is directly proportional to how much you dread the task. The more you dread the task, the more energy you will spend trying to complete the task. Daniel Kahneman, the author of *Thinking Fast and Slow*, best describes this phenomenon.

"An effort of will or self-control is tiring; if you have had to force yourself to do something, you are less willing or less able to exert self-control when the next challenge comes around."

This means that, if you spend your time on one task, you will have less energy to complete the next one. So how do you escape this energy-draining trap? According to Kahneman, you do it by exerting better self-control and managing your efforts. As we saw in earlier chapters, this self-control or willpower is a finite resource, and its conservation should be the main focus here. This is where the Law of Least Effort comes in. Let's take a more in-depth look at what it entails.

The Law of Least Effort

Also known as Zipf's Law, Zipf's Principle of Least Effort, and the path of least resistance, the premise of this law is pretty simple. If something can be done in multiple ways, the one that uses the least effort is always better. This principle is a deterministic description of human behavior. It not only appeals to the fundamentally lazy part of us (our subconscious that loves doing things on autopilot), but it also provides a more efficient way of doing things, which, in turn, means we still end up with the same results but with less effort.

It also states that everything in life has a flow; struggling against this flow will only cause you undue stress and pain. A good example of something that follows the path of least resistance is water. If you poured a glass of water on the floor and watched it flow, it follows the path with the fewest obstacles. It doesn't push or struggle against furniture but rather goes around any obstacles in its way.

Objectively and subjectively, we link effort to greater value. A precious gem such as a diamond is valuable because it's scarce and requires a great deal of effort to find. You would tend to value a goal more if you faced numerous obstacles to overcome it. For instance, on your journey to change your habits, you might value your new habits more if you failed several times while trying to create them. Generally, we can agree that effort is a positive and praiseworthy value.

That said, not all effort yields good results. For instance, you can do math by hand or use a calculator. However, doing it by hand requires more effort, and you are prone to making more errors. In such a case, the amount of effort invested in the action isn't proportional to the results; in fact, it is a waste of energy.

The most important thing you must understand is that this principle doesn't seek to eliminate the difficulty in a task nor does it encourage us to take the easy way out. It's not being carefree or too relaxed and not caring about what happens. Instead, it focuses on finding ways to reduce the amount of effort and energy used to complete a task. This way, you have enough energy to tackle the next task. The law simply aims to help you reduce your work expenditure over time.

Even with the increased efficiency, there will be difficulties. After all, you are adopting a new position, and you will still need to use up a bit of energy. These obstacles are present in everyday tasks, and sometimes we require a lot of energy to solve them. Even then, things don't go our way, and it can leave us feeling overwhelmed and disappointed. This makes it even harder to face the same challenges the next day.

This is where we end up struggling with our total resistance to continue and the obligation to do so. Having wasted so much emotional energy in this struggle and still not having achieved anything, we are left frustrated. The work we are doing is not proportional to what we are achieving, but we cannot abandon it either.

Practicing the Law of Least Effort

Sticking to the book's main theme, how can we apply this law in our everyday lives? Just like water, we need to find our own path of least resistance. Here are a few steps to help you find this path.

Prepare yourself

Before you start, you need to make 3 commitments:

- Acceptance, which, in this case, means taking the good along with the bad. We are more accepting of good things but often have a hard time dealing with the bad stuff. For instance, if you got a promotion today, you'd be thrilled, even though it meant more work; but, if you lost a job you have loathed working at, you would be distraught.

In such a case, you need to accept the bad just as you accepted the god. Rather than dwelling on the hurt and despair, you need to accept what happened and move on. That said, you should give yourself some time to deal with these emotions; after all, suppressing them will only lead to worse outcomes. When applying the law of least effort, acceptance means acknowledging what's going on but not sitting around and letting life pass you by.

- Take responsibility. Practicing this law doesn't provide you with an excuse not to put any effort into things.

It's not a pass to not try, but rather it means accepting the situation you are in, taking responsibility for your life, and taking real action to go in the direction you want to.

- Lastly, surrender; just like the water, you need to surrender yourself to the flow or process. The biggest cause of anxiety and stress in life is the desire to control everything that happens. You think that if you control the outcomes, you are going to be okay. However, life is unpredictable, and many times, you will find that you have very little, if any control over what happens. This desire to control things will cause resistance, which slows down your progress and results in unnecessary pain.

Resist the urge to react

There are different types of people in the world, and there's a very high chance you might not like or get along with some of them. For instance, they talk too loudly or chew with their mouths open. Whatever the reason, responding with negativity to such randomness will only leave you feeling bad and use up way too much energy. To help you resist such urges, imagine yourself inside an invisible bubble that only lets positive energy in and shields you from the negative energy.

Emulate nature

If you are having a hard time giving up control, spending some time in nature can help you let go of this rigidity you have held onto for so long. It allows you to relax and open yourself up to different possibilities.

Accept your emotions and mood

Practicing the law of least effort is meant to help you conserve as much of your energy as possible. Having good energy reserves means you will be in a positive mood. However, sometimes you might not be feeling so chipper and you can't help it. It's normal to have bad days and to feel both good and bad emotions. However, trying to force yourself to feel happy when you are feeling sad only puts more focus on your bad mood.

Rather than trying to fix it and get back to being positive, sometimes it's okay to surrender to the bad day; do what you can to take care of yourself and try again tomorrow. This is a great point to remember when you are working on any of the areas we covered in the book, such as loving yourself more or changing behaviors and habits.

Be present

Lastly, work on being present in the moment. Another reason we are always so anxious is that we are worried about things that haven't happened or might not happen. For instance, you might worry that your fiancé's family won't like you when you haven't even met them. This means you experience the stress of meeting them twice, first in your mind and second in reality. However, if the meeting never happens, you stress over nothing.

Life is full of unknowns and stressing over them won't change the outcome; in fact, it weakens your ability to face them. If you are anxious about something you can't control, you won't be present in the moment and might miss out on everything that's going on. Additionally, learning to be present not only reduces stress but can also help you find other ways to get things done. The more present you are, the more things you see and observe. This new information can even help you find an alternative way to solve a problem you have.

Practicing the law of least effort is an act of trust; trust that no matter what happens, it's for the greater good. Even bad, hurtful experiences hold some significance because their lessons will be pivotal to your growth. Remember, you cannot stop the waves, but you can learn how to surf.

Being Content and Accepting Change

If you would like to be happier and more content in life, you have to learn how to embrace change. But aren't these two things opposites? Many times, people have presented contentment and change as opposing ideas. This is because, stereotypically, a content person is shown as someone who is satisfied with their life and never wants more than what they have. In this narrative, they still live in the same house they did as kids, wear the same clothes, use the same gadgets, and so on.

However, this is a flawed concept of what being content means. It states that we should be happy with our lives as they are and never try to change or improve them. Change, however, is an inevitable part of life. Humans are designed to evolve and change according to their surroundings, which means that nothing in life is static. For instance, to survive, we have to learn how to adapt; if we do not, we die.

Often, when told to choose between maintaining the status quo or making a change, doing the latter often results in a happier life in the long run. But this is easier said than done. Making a change is scary, and this fear has left many people living unhappy lives because they fear the unknown that comes with change. How many people do you know who still go to jobs they loath every day? How many people are dating narcissists, knowing they are no good but being unable to shed their fear of being alone?

Fear of change is irrational; however, this doesn't mean it's not real to the person experiencing it. For instance, someone dating a narcissist is trapped in an unhealthy relationship because they are convinced that if they leave, no one will love them. But think about it, can they truly be unlovable? Contrary to what they think, they are loved but have a hard time seeing it because they don't love themselves. For this person to have a truly happy life, they have to come to accept who they are and be ready to fight for it. However, such a change can be a bit overwhelming.

Change, whether big or small, has been found to be a major cause of depression. While it is not solely responsible for causing depression, it is a major contributing factor. This is because change begets change, and even minute changes can affect your happiness. Take, for instance, moving to a new city. This means you need to get a new place and job. This means meeting new people in a place that's unfamiliar to you. You can see how everything starts to unravel.

So how can we still be content and happy through change?

Finding the answer to this question means embarking on a personal journey of self-discovery. The first step entails dealing with your fears.

- **Look at your fears more objectively**—a lot of the fear induced by change is irrational. You spend so much time worrying over hypotheticals that might not happen. For instance, after leaving an unhealthy relationship, it's easy to get lost in thoughts of never finding love again. These, in turn, keep you from opening yourself up to the many opportunities you have of meeting great people, thus feeding into the flawed logic that there's something wrong with you.

However, if you took the time to look at things more objectively, you would get a more realistic picture of what will or won't happen. Think about the big picture here—what does closing yourself off to others really get you? Afterward, you can use your best judgment to determine if what you fear will come true. This also lets you get out of your head where things often seem a lot worse than they really are.

- **Evaluate your definition of happiness**—before you start dwelling on how change has messed up your idea of happiness, you need to define what happiness means to you. What does it take to make you truly happy? What needs to happen for you to be truly happy? What is your happiness recipe? For example, happiness to you might be spending time with loved ones.

This exercise will force you to truly evaluate yourself and you may discover that the change you are experiencing does not affect your happiness.

Let's say you lose your job; this can be quite distressing, especially if you have a family; however, it presents you with a great chance to spend more time with your family while you are in between jobs. While this is a distressing experience, because your happiness is defined by spending time with family, you remain happy and resolve any negative feelings you may have been having.

- **Change your happiness standards**—let's say happiness for you is making six figures and living the high life or traveling the world. However, if you don't have a job or money, it's hard to travel the world or earn six figures. In your current situation where you have lost your job, such happiness standards are unrealistic and are bound to make you feel dissatisfied with life.

In such a case, you might have to dig deep and redefine what happiness is to you. Making a lot of money made you happy before, however now that you have lost your job or quit, is it still your definition of happiness? Hanging on to unrealistic definitions of happiness will make it harder for you to embrace change or even achieve happiness. You will be stuck thinking of all the things you would have if you made all that money, making you resentful of your current situation.

After some deep soul searching, you might find that making a lot of money was only important because you wanted to provide for your loved ones. If you change your happiness definition from making a lot of money to providing for your loved ones, you might find the change a lot more practical and manageable.

- **Count your blessings**—a simple way to be happier is appreciating everything you have. Whenever you find yourself feeling unsatisfied with your life, take a moment to count all the good things in your life. Be happy that you have a loving family, health, and a job, among others. You can be grateful for so many things, and focusing on them will make you happier.

A good way to get this done is by showing the people in your life that you appreciate them. Giving a hug or spending time with them can go a long way to showing your gratitude. Counting your blessings also includes learning to enjoy the simple things. Rather than focusing on trying to get expensive things and spending lots of money on things, you can learn to enjoy free stuff. Not to sound trite, but the things that make us most happy are often free.

- **Lastly, let go of attachments**—to live a truly content life, you have to learn how to let go of things. In the example we used earlier about moving to a new city, you are essentially leaving the life you had in your hometown, and it can be quite hard. If you don't let go of your attachments, you will have a hard time getting your new life together. If you are still too hung up on a relationship you had, you will have a hard time finding someone new, which means that you will likely remain miserable.

However, this is easier said than done. After all, these attachments are important to you and the connection might be very strong. Nonetheless, if you have been following the steps we have gone through, you now understand that happiness comes from within. You are the main determining factor when it comes to your own happiness. That isn't to say that these attachments are not important; however, it's important to prioritize your happiness.

Once you start accepting that happiness comes from inside you and that change cannot hinder your happiness, you will be able to face anything that comes your way. The key to being content is setting a standard of happiness that is independent of external factors. Note that implementing these steps and achieving contentment is a slow process, but don't forget you are still changing and actively striving for happiness.

Final Words: Making it Last

IT HAS BEEN QUITE a long ride and a lot has been said. We've discussed how to handle stress, show yourself more self-love, deal with change, form new habits, work on your willpower, and more. Every single topic is meant to help us get through the everyday struggles we face.

The tips and advice included here are meant to act as a guide. They are intended to help you remain standing when life pulls the rug right from under you. In life, the chances of being caught unprepared more than once are pretty high. Remember, change is inevitable; in fact, it's pretty much a constant, so you have to learn to adapt to it.

Achieving happiness and inner peace in all their elusive glory takes hard work, but you can do it. You are going to fail and get disappointed many more times than you would like, but if you keep at it, you'll make it. My job here is simply to remind you of that. The trick to finding contentment and living a stress-free, happy life is changing your perspective—the way you think and feel. Once you take this step, grab hold of it, and watch as your life changes for the better.

www.ingramcontent.com/pod-product-compliance
Lightning Source LLC
Chambersburg PA
CBHW061501250726
48657CB00005B/1688